THE HEALTHY NUMBERS

VOLUME 1

"EASY GUIDE TO HEALTHIER MIDDLE EASTERN CUISINE"

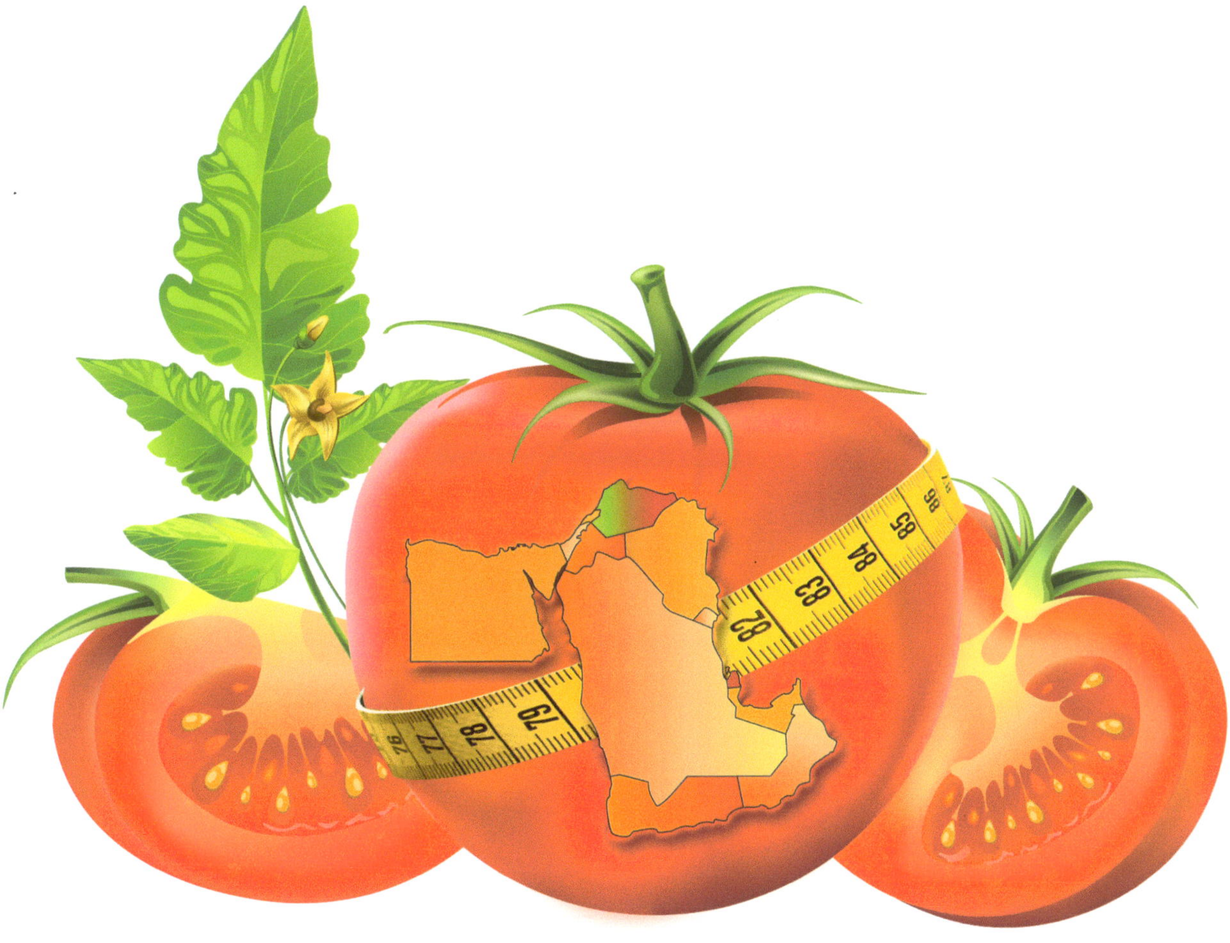

THE HEALTHY NUMBERS

VOLUME 1

"EASY GUIDE TO HEALTHIER MIDDLE EASTERN CUISINE"

Racha Sankar

VJ

PUBLISHING HOUSE, LLC.

United States of America

Published by: VJ Publishing House, LLC

Printed in the United States of America

First Printing, 2013 July

VJ Publishing House, LLC.
320 S. Flamingo Rd., Suite #305
Pembroke Pines, FL 33027

www.VJPUBLISHINGHOUSE.com

ISBN: 978-1-939236-01-2
Library of Congress Control Number: 1-962625766

Photographer: Tarek Alwawi (Syria)

Creative Graphic Designer: Gabriel Zanabria of Printing Nation USA, LLC.

Illustrator Designer: Ruba Dehneh (Syria)

DEDICATIONS

Dedication

My dedication is to you
To the *City of Jasmine*
To where I was born
To streets I walked on
To water springs I drank from
To the people of Jasmine

To every blood drop that fell everywhere
To every house bombed and destroyed
To every Syrian crying for their beloved ones
To every child being harmed day after day
To every Mother suffering for her kids
To every Father struggling to bring the bread
To every family spending days and nights under gunshots and bombs

To every Syrian who could not handle the stress
To every Syrian who packed and left
To schools and shelters that children were forced to live in
To every Syrian helping others and never-mind the risk of attempts
To every Syrian who doesn't know what's going to happen next
To every Syrian aiming to rebuild and reassess
To the tears of Syrian children
To the sorrow of Syrians' eyes
To the depression of Syrians everywhere

Here,I leave a Syrian fingerprint
I wish I could have left it somewhere else
Where everyone would feel safe and at rest
To all of you, my beloved Syrians
I share my book in the darkest moments that we are going through
I pray to God that our Syria will stand and shine soon
Sooner than anyone would expect
Always, Racha

Syrians' Eyes

What tyrannies did to you
They killed you or they slaughtered you
With gunshots they profaned you
With tanks' smoke they offended you
The dust of weapons overwhelmed you
They made your people immigrants
They made your kids orphans
They murdered your youth

Syrians'eyes are running out of tears
Mothers and daughters are crying for Fathers and peers
Men are shouting how to feed their kids, they are so dear
They did not care about your infants, no God's fear

Syria, you are the memories of love for us
Memories of days under olive trees and between wheat spikes
Memories of days by Bardah River, the pleasure of childhood's bikes
Memories of our days by Al Fejah Springs, the joyful water no one dislikes
What about the Jasmine? We cry you and the fragrance that everywhere flies
&
Kassioun Mountain; it overlooks the historical Damascus, hurtfully it cries

Syria, please stay strong
You are being hurt; trust me it's not for long
Syrians, have faith, peace will return
Syrians, have faith, soon, we are back to re-bond
We are for our Syria, where we are proud to belong

Always, Racha

TO THE MEMORY OF

Hayat Alsoufi

"Grandmother"
1933-2013

I never thought that I would change my acknowledgment at the last
moment because of losing someone so dear,
my Grandma**, **Teta Hayat
I did not have the chance to hand this book to you, as you were
waiting to see my final work and always praying for me
***Teta Hayat**, the fragrance of your advice and the aroma of your*
prayers are always the blessing that will help me Stand
May your soul rest in peace
I love you and you will always be in my prayers...

Foreword

The inception of this book was not planned rather evolved as a result of Racha Sankar's RPh, D. experiences as a nutritionist working with medical professionals while in Syria. As her professor in the Dietetics and Nutrition program at Florida International University, she asked me for advice on how to put a book together. Honestly, I knew the process was going to be very long and never thought that it would one day be published.

She had to document all of the traditional food recipes and planned as to how they can be made more nutritious and better without losing taste and appearance. My advice was to test all of the traditional recipes and modify them to reduce calories and fat in her kitchen. She did test all of them, and had family and friends taste and verify that the new recipes were acceptable. The next step was to make the nutritional analysis of the traditional recipes versus the healthy recipes to compare them. The food exchanges, portion sizes of foods, and balanced meal combinations were also determined. The final step was to prepare all the recipes again in order to photograph them for the book. Thus became the book you have in your hands.

The recipes in this book are presented side by side and with nutritional value to follow. This is not only a cook book, but also a nutritional education book. Readers and users of this book will learn about nutrition without ever knowing that they are. I was happy to be a part of this process as an Advisor.

I endorse the content and information provided on nutrition to be sound and accurate. As a professor of nutrition for 30 years, I rarely endorse products of commercial value. This is truly intended to help people to eat better, and be healthy, not a commercial venture. This book can be used by anyone with Middle Eastern taste or adventurous individuals who may like to try Middle Eastern cooking with healthy recipes.

Fatma G. Huffman PhD, RD
Professor and Chair
Department of Dietetics and Nutrition
Florida International University

TABLE OF CONTENTS

RECIPES

Grains:

Meat:

Dairy Products:

Vegetables:

Dear Reader,

I would like to take the time to thank you for reading my book. While you join my nutrition journey with Middle Eastern foods, I want to share some thoughts and beliefs with you. I will be honest and whisper that despite the modification of recipes that took place in this book; the goal was always to save Middle Eastern traditional cuisine and not to change it overtime. Since we have to cope with the technology and cross cultural food invasion, we open the door to high prevalence of obesity, chronic diseases we have, and the more our children forget the taste of the Middle Eastern foods. Children of today are parents of tomorrow, and food preferences are acquired overtime. Most of today's mothers do not cook on Fridays, because today's grandmothers raised them teaching that Friday is the day for relaxation and eating out. Ask yourself, how many times you bring fast food to your family in a week? Then ask how many times your parents brought you fast food in a month 10 years ago?

We save our health and tradition when we cook at home and go back to food habits our parents taught us. We acquired these habits from our parents, and we should not want our children to eat fast food everyday when they become parents. No! No! and No! to any cross cultural food habit that destroys the health of our bodies and eliminates the joyful and tasty recipes of Middle Eastern cuisine.

We have to cope with technology improvements but that does not require us to forget our health. We cannot ignore the fact of the importance of the dishwasher, laundry machines, and many other technologies in saving time and efficiency. However, exercise and recipe modifications go here. Exercise is the only replacement for physical activities that females used to do at home. With all the benefits personal computers bring to everyone's life, it has the worst impact on our health. Most men spend eight hours a day doing sedentary (desk) work a day. Medical experts describes this as a lack of physical activity and puts one at a higher risk of every type of chronic disease. Still, 60 minutes of exercise is considered "healthy", but it must be combined with dietary guidelines. Again, exercise and recipe modifications are the only replacements here. If we are forced to cope with technology, we have to accept the fact of modifying recipes and exercising to protect ourselves against any future epidemic disorders and obesity with its related diseases.

Mothers, your kitchen is your kingdom, where you reduce the incidence of every disease you and your family members are at risk of. Rest assure, the more you cook at home, the healthier your children will be. Always remember, you are the key to your family's health. Your food selections determine the health status of your family. Mothers with healthy lifestyles have children with high *Healthy Numbers*. Think twice before you eat out or before you order fast foods. The healthy diet leads to healthy bodies and to healthy brains. Thus, consider teaching healthy eating guidelines as one of your responsibilities towards your children.

I'm pretty sure that I will not succeed at making everyone quit eating western and junk foods, but I'm so confident that I will convince many people to cut down on consumption of these foods, or to eat them in moderation.

I truly hope that my nutrition book is able to help you make a serious decision to move towards a healthier lifestyle. Always remember, that a single step forward is a great improvement in your and your family's health.

My door is open to listen to your comments and to provide answers to your questions. Your constructive observations will always be considered.

Sincerely,

Racha

Nutrition is my Lego game; it is never a picture puzzle!

I do not believe that nutrition convinces you to eat what you don't like to eat, but nutrition is able to provide you with healthier alternatives you will definitely enjoy. Pieces of picture puzzles must be placed selectively, but pieces of Legos are more entertaining because you decide what you want to create.

Introduction

The rate of obesity is increasing worldwide. The Middle East is not immune to these increases. In fact, in Middle Eastern countries the rate of obesity is much higher than western countries. The Middle East and the Gulf areas traditionally have a healthy cuisine in which foods can be combined to include all of the macro and micronutrients in a balanced way. If we were living 20-30 years ago, no cuisine would be healthier than Middle Eastern cuisine. Nevertheless, different factors had negative influences on the health of the people living in this region. In contrast to belief, food consumption plays a major role in the increasing rate of obesity and related diseases. The improved food industry, fast food invasion, and advanced technologies are the main factors that led to a sedentary lifestyle, lack of physical activity, and over consumption of empty calorie foods daily. No wonder, a great increase in the rate of obesity and chronic diseases is seen and diagnosed amongst different aged groups from the Middle East and the Gulf region.

Twenty to thirty years ago, obesity was not a major health concern. Diabetes, hypertension, and hypercholesterolemia were diseases found in the elderly population. People rarely heard of a young man dying from a heart attack, a child being diagnosed with type 2 diabetes, a man in his thirties being on kidney dialysis, a teenager going under bariatric surgery, a 25-year old woman being diagnosed with osteoporosis, and commonly; people being constipated or having digestive problems.

Calorie counting, fad diets, juice diets, bad and good foods, aggressive exercise, weight loss pills, fat burners, and herbal remedies are the most common trends amongst people living in this region. These trendy diets are used in order to eliminate nutritional related health issues such as constipation, high lipid profiles, high blood pressure, high blood sugar, and weight gain. In reality, no health professional can recommend or guarantee any of the previous trendy diets, if it is not combined with lifestyle changes. The miracle solution people seek from any trendy approach can be found in the traditional Middle Eastern cuisine rather than spending money and time to reach impermanent solutions with no certain health benefits.

In the last 30 years, we have been living in a world of technology explosion. Unfortunately, the food industry, fast food invasion and technology developments are reasons for poor health outcomes.

Developments within the fast food industries makes it easier for people to make wrong choices in food selections, especially snacks. People are easily lost among those amazingly packed biscuits, appealing chocolate bars, colorful cereal boxes, multi-flavored potato chips, and wide range of soft drinks and sodas; besides the microwavable and pre-cooked foods. Nuts and dried fruits are healthy snacks that contribute nutrients and fiber to our diet. They are being diced with sugar and fat by the food industry to increase their appeal to young children. Nuts are rich in healthy fat, polyunsaturated fatty acid, but when they are coated with butter or chocolate, saturated fat (bad fat) will be dominant. The food industry also soaks dried fruits with chocolate, sugar and high fructose corn syrup converting them from high fiber snacks to high caloric snacks.

Moreover, the introduction of numerous foods and artificial flavors and many types of juices makes nutrition experts think carefully before recommending juice to their patients and clients. Different juices have different manufacturing processes, different additives, different nutritional values and most are not nutritionally sound due to high sugar content.

The processed foods are always packed with misleading food labels that claim health benefits. Consumers are made to believe the effect of these sneaky advertisements. Misleading labels such as fiber-enriched or cholesterol free attract people and make them unintentionally consume large quantities of these products. When people adopt the habits of consuming processed foods, they reduce the consumption of healthy foods. Children acquire the same habits, because parents are the strongest role model for their children. For instance, whole wheat bread is replaced with oatmeal biscuits and cereals. Biscuits and cereals contain less fiber and more calories with less satiety feeling than same sized portions of whole wheat bread. Food advertisements totally change the real image of products leading people to make poor food choices, particularly children. For example, when a cartoon character eats potato chips that are cholesterol free, children will love to eat the product with their parental approval. In reality, potato chips are high in hydrogenated oil that worsens the overall lipid profile and is a main reason for cholesterol accumulation on veins and arteries.

A visit to any food court in shopping malls supports the invasion of fast foods into lifestyles of people living in the Middle East and the Gulf regions. Their menus include burgers, breaded meat and chicken, cheese-sauced french fries, and mayonnaise-dressed fresh salads. Sandwiches are filled with cheese and sauces, and meals are combined with french fries, sauces, and soda. Fast food restaurants are everywhere with the option of drive thru or home delivery, factors that promote their consumption. People acquire the taste of fast foods as it is time saving. Fast foods used to be the foods for holidays; unfortunately, now they are the foods of everyday. The more people eat fast foods or eat out, the more they experience digestive problems over time. People might not realize the bad influences of fast foods on the day of consumption, but eventually they experience a big belly, constant bloating and constipation. They probably relate those digestive problems to aging or to innocent foods they rarely consume. In fact, the fast foods are also the main reasons for high lipid profile and weight gain. Any fast food meal contains less fiber and many more calories than same sized portion of traditional foods.

Dishwashers, laundry machines; steam irons; television; computers and transportation development are reasons for the lack of physical activities particularly in women's lifestyles. Computer, internet, and online businesses are other reasons that have a greater negative influence on overall physical activities, particularly in men. Children are now helping their parents in solving any technology issues such as mobile applications and computer programs. The introduction of electronics into children's lifestyles might have expanded the horizons of education, but it is an essential reason for their physical inactivity and obesity.

Although these changes might not be measurable at the moment, the frequent exposure to those factors is the main reason for the change of people's eating habits and nutritional behaviors in the Middle East and the Gulf areas. Thus, it widens the extent of obesity and its related chronic diseases to different aged groups including children, adolescence, and middle aged people. Different studies established in different Middle East and Gulf countries demonstrated high prevalence of chronic diseases amongst the middle age population. For instance, a random sample population study in United Arab Emirates showed that the rate of diabetes among 30-64 years old participants was 29%, and 24.2% had pre diabetes [25]. A study aimed to indicate the prevalence of coronary risks among healthy Kuwaiti adults found that one-third of Kuwaiti population is obese as well as 4.7% of Kuwaiti females are morbidly obese [28]. Again, a study supporting the previous findings showed that prevalence of type 2 diabetes among Kuwaiti men younger than 55 years old was 49.5%, and it is 56.9% among men of all ages [3]. In Saudi Arabia, multiple studies indicated the high prevalence of obesity among women, men, and children [5, 22]. Accordingly, another study in Saudi Arabia stated that there is14.2% obese men and 23.6% obese women [4]. This study also demonstrated that the overweight prevalence is 30.7% in men, and it is 28.4% in women [4]. Studies concluded that 10.8% of the preschool Saudi children are obese [2]. The cross-sectional national epidemiological household survey for 12,071 Saudi children showed that there are 10.7% overweight boys and 12.7% overweight girls [10]. A study aimed to indicate the change in obesity for prevalence during the past 10 years in Jordan stated that the incorporation of western style foods into Mediterranean diet was associated with obesity [14]. Another finding demonstrated higher risks of heart disease, cerebro-vascular disease, and cancer among Palestinians due to consumption of western style foods [13]. The result of a cross sectional survey with 2,104 of the Lebanese showed that 30% of boys were overweight and obese, 19.3% girls were obese and overweight, 72% men were obese and overweight, and 68.2% of women were overweight and obese [26]. The poor results of the self-rating health survey conducted with Syrian women suggested the need of more interventions and lifestyle changes in order to improve the health status of Syrian women [8]. In Aleppo, the 2nd largest city in Syria, the prevalence of obesity was 46.4% in women and 28.8% in men [19]. A study indicated that the prevalence of obesity in urban areas of Egypt is 56% and it is 44% in rural areas [18]. A large research reviewed of 51 studies included 267,537 participants in the Middle Eastern countries found that the overall prevalence of obesity was 24.5%, type 2 diabetes was 10.5%, and hypertension was 21.7% [20]. The rate of every chronic disease is increasing; and most people with chronic diseases are either overweight or obese. Twenty years ago, the genetic factors were the main risk factors for any chronic diseases; today lifestyle is the critical key in chronic disease development.

If people do not take healthier steps towards healthy eating and physical activity, obesity and chronic diseases will continue to increase in this region. It is effortless to this population to lessen the rate of obesity and chronic diseases if mothers and fathers of today implement what their parents taught them and how their parental lifestyles used to be. If people of this region go backwards to their traditions, great steps forward will be recognized in their health and wellness. Since people get accustomed to western foods, and world technology development is essential; the people must follow guidelines to improve their low health scores. Healthier lifestyle is the key, and moderation plays the most important role. Adopting a healthy lifestyle is a series of actions people have to consider everyday. However, moderation is necessary when people have to break the guidelines of their healthy lifestyles.

The principles of a healthy lifestyle are good eating habits and physical activity. Good eating habits include a balanced daily diet. Breakfast is an essential meal, half of main meals must be vegetable and fruits, four fiber-rich small meals, a serving from the milk group, 8-12 cups of water, and monounsaturated fat and polyunsaturated fat are alternatives to saturated fat.

People face different barriers to healthy lifestyles such as (food preferences, work environment, social relationships, holidays, access to healthful meals, inadequate cooking skills, advertised foods, computer use, television viewing and lack of nutritional skills). Generally, the greatest obstacle to a healthy lifestyle is the misconception of it. People associate healthy eating patterns to hospital foods, weight loss programs, and eating behaviors of nutritional experts. They also tend to relate fast foods and eating out events to pleasure and love. Unfortunately, people are reluctant to believe that they have to follow health-promoting guidelines everyday, and they partially break any of the guidelines when they cannot handle the situation. The swing in weight loss and weight gain is such a common example to support the misconception of a healthy lifestyle. When people practice the nutritional skills of weight maintenance, they probably live healthier lifestyles. In other words, when people follow a programmed diet to lose weight, to relieve constipation, to balance blood sugar, or to improve lipid profiles, they experience satisfying results. The results are not reached by following trendy-overdoing programmed diets. The realistic lifelong solutions are to live a healthy lifestyles and to maintain new eating habits. When people are fully convinced to adopt healthful guidelines on a daily basis, obstacles will be clear to them and multiple solutions to every obstacle will be available. For example, when a person does not have breakfast because he goes to work early but decides to make healthy steps forward, taking a sandwich with a serving of fresh vegetables to work will be a reasonable solution; having the breakfast prepare in the work cafeteria is another realistic solution, or waking up earlier to have breakfast is also a doable solution.

The implementation of a healthy lifestyle requires an individual's determination and commitment. An individual has to identify their undesirable eating habits, barriers to healthy eating habits, solutions to overcome barriers, and several healthier eating habits to follow. The importance of physical activity to reduce risk factors of diseases and improve overall health should also be incorporated into a daily routine.

Moderation is necessary when eating out or consuming high caloric foods such as fast foods, chocolate bars, and desserts. Wherever, whatever, and whenever we eat, portion control is the most important skill every individual has to master in order to have health and wellness.

This book is a guide to those who want to eat healthier, to lose weight, and to avoid or reduce risk of chronic disease. It contains recipes of common Middle Eastern dishes tested by the author herself under a controlled environment.

This book includes recipes modification in order to reduce calories and to increase nutritional benefits of foods. Nutritional analysis, calories from macronutrients, fiber content, food exchanges, meal combinations, and portion sizes are reported. Comparisons between traditional recipes and healthy recipes are tested and also documented to help the reader try healthier recipes for improving their health.

Glossary & Instructions

Calorie is the unit of energy provided by foods; it is the amount of energy required to raise one gram of water by one degree celsius.

Micronutrients are the vitamins and minerals that are necessary for the body reactions and functions. Different micronutrients have different functions in the body. (Thiamin, riboflavin, niacin, vitamin B6, vitamin B12, folate, vitamin C, vitamin A, vitamin E, calcium, iron, magnesium, potassium, zinc, and sodium).

Macronutrients are large molecules that provide the energy to the body, fat, protein, and carbohydrate.

Fat is one of the macronutrients and has different functions in the body. 1 gram of fat provides 9 calories. Fat is classified into healthy fat and bad fat according to their chemical structures and functions. Monounsaturated fat, polyunsaturated fat, Omega-3-fatty acid (Omega-3-FA), and Omega-6-fatty acid (Omega-6-FA) have positive influence on lipid profiles, blood vessels and heart health. In contrast to saturated fat, trans fat, and cholesterol are the bad types of fat that have negative influence on lipid profile when over-consumed.

Protein is one of the macronutrients and has different functions in the body. 1 gram of protein provides 4 calories.

Carbohydrate is one of the macronutrients and the main source of energy. 1 gram of carbohydrate provides 4 calories.

Calories from Macronutrients:

The comparison between the macronutrient contents of the traditional recipe and the healthy recipe shows that Middle Eastern recipes are high in fat compared to protein and carbohydrate and lack complex carbohydrate. The modification of recipes balances the percentages of calories provided by the 3 macronutrients in order to improve the nutritional quality of the Middle Eastern foods. The goal of the modification is to reduce calories from fat and substitute them for calories from protein and carbohydrate. Also, it aims to increase the consumption of complex carbohydrate and to change the types of fat to healthier fat.

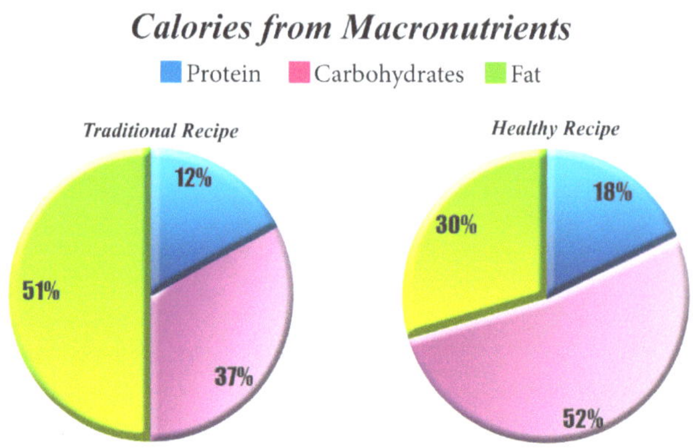

% Fiber intake Compared to Average Daily Needs:

Fiber is an important nutrient in the body; it has multiple health benefits. Fiber eliminates most of the digestive problems in addition to its role in preventing a wide range of diseases. The human body lacks the enzymes that digest fiber; it does not provide calories and delays the digestion process resulting in a delayed hunger. It also slows the absorption of glucose into the bloodstream after each meal and creates a bulk in the colon to eliminate constipation and bloating. Most Middle Eastern recipes are low in fiber content; an addition to every meal is required. The modification aims to increase fiber content and to maintain appeal and flavor of the foods.

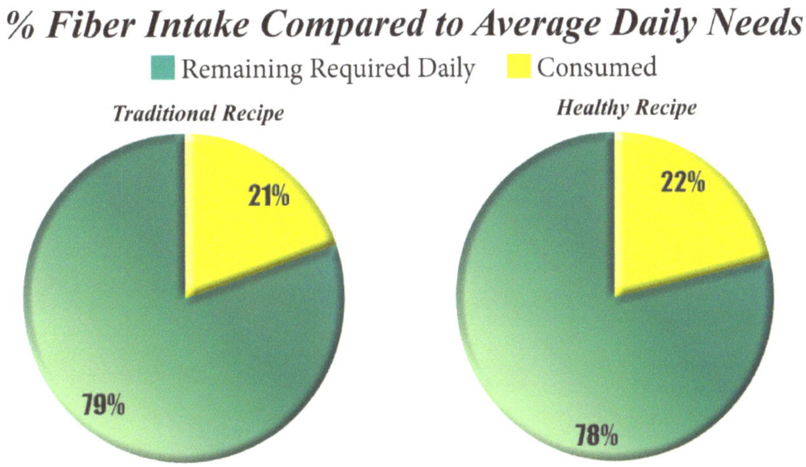

Food Exchange for meals:

The food exchange of the recipes has a vital role in diabetes management since diabetic individuals have to follow certain nutritional guidelines to keep blood glucose at maintenance level. The food exchange also helps individuals develop their own weight loss meal plans. Thus, the food exchanges for every dish are provided as well as the food exchanges for the healthy meal combination are determined.

Food Exchanges for every dish:

Number of Exchanges Per Serving: 1 Cup

Traditional Recipe	Healthy Recipe
4 1/2 fat exchange (PUFA)	1 1/4 fat exchange (MUFA)
1 grain exchange	1 grain exchange
3/4 starch exchange	2/3 starch exchange
1 3/4 meat exchange (3/4 very lean, 1 medium fat)	1 1/3 meat exchange (2/3 very lean, 3/4 lean)

Food Exchange for the healthy meal combination:

Healthy Recipe (Calorie Controlled & Content Balanced)	**Number of Exchanges in a Balanced Meal**
Men	**Men**
2 1/2 cups of burghul be al-tamatum 3 cups of green salad-drizzled with olive oil 1 cup of lowfat ayran	2 1/2 grain exchange 5 non-starchy vegetable exchange 4 3/4 fat exchange 1 milk exchange
Women	**Women**
1 1/2 cups of burghul be al-tamatum 1 1/2 cups of green salad-drizzled with olive oil 1 cup of lowfat ayran	1 1/2 grain exchange 2 3/4 non-starchy vegetable exchange 2 1/2 fat exchange 1 milk exchange

The table of the nutritional analysis of the traditional recipes and the healthy recipes:

The table of the nutritional analysis shows the calorie contents and nutrient contents in the same portions of the traditional recipes and the healthy recipes. It helps individuals determine their calorie consumption when dieting, and it shows the nutritional values added to the healthy recipes in numbers when compared to the traditional recipes.

Nutrient Content	Traditional Recipe	Healthy Recipe
Portion	1 cup	1 cup
Weight (g)	244	206
Kilocalories (kcal)	428.41	246.99
Protein (g)	13.75	12
Carbohydrate (g)	40.7	33.69
Fat (g)	24.94	8.6
Saturated Fat (g)	4.21	1.6
Monounsaturated Fat (g)	6.59	5.5
Polyunsaturated Fat (g)	12.46	1.1
Trans Fatty Acid (g)	0.29	0.1
Cholesterol (g)	16.7	14.9
Omega-6 Linoleic (g)	11.92	0.65
Omega-3 Linolenic (g)	0.3	0.15
Fiber (g)	7.59	8.2
Sugar (g)	2.17	2.4
Water (L)	3.7	21.3
Thiamin (mg)	0.24	0.14
Riboflavin (mg)	0.17	0.11
Niacin (mg)	4.31	3.8
Vitamin B6 (mg)	0.27	0.35
Vitamin B12 (mcg)	0.533	0.54
Folate (DFE) mcg	15.4	28.6
Vitamin C (mg)	25.11	24.4
Vitamin D (mcg)	0	0
Vitamin A (RAE) (mcg)	77.44	0.1
Vitamin E (mg)	3.49	0.78
Calcium (mg)	37.39	33.9
Iron (mg)	2.9	2.16
Magnesium (mg)	99.7	94.23
Potassium (mg)	443.22	583
Zinc (mg)	2.32	2.6
Sodium (mg)	60	25.4

Recommended portion sizes and meal combination:

The recommended portion sizes of the traditional recipes are controlled to meet an average amount of calories that must be consumed in a meal for men and women.

When the recommended portion sizes of the healthy recipes vary to meet the nutritional requirements for balanced meals and to meet an average amount of calories that must be consumed in a meal for men and women.

The meal combination of the traditional recipes and the healthy recipes vary according to the traditional norms of how foods are served in the region.

Recommended Portion Sizes & Meal Combinations

Traditional Recipe (Calorie Controlled)	Healthy Recipe (Calorie Controlled & Content Balanced)
Men 1 1/4 cups of burghul be al-tamatum 1 1/4 cups of traditional green salad	**Men** 2 1/2 cups of burghul be al-tamatum 3 cups of green salad-drizzled with olive oil 1 cup of lowfat ayran
Women 2/3 cup of burghul be al-tamatum 1 cup of traditional green salad	**Women** 1 1/2 cups of burghul be al-tamatum 1 1/2 cups of green salad-drizzled with olive oil 1 cup of lowfat ayran

Obesity Prevalence in Middle East and Gulf Areas among Children and Adolescents

Country	Obesity Prevalence	Year of Study	Age Range	Reference Number
Syria	27.50%	2009	15-18	21
Palastine	16.50%	2009	12-18	7
Jordan	25%	2009	2-18	15
Egypt	39%	2006	11-19	24
Lebanon	44.50%	2010	14-18	12
Saudi Arabia	34.50%	2010	5-18	9
Yemen	8%	2005	2-5	27
Oman	32.40%	2004	15-18	23
Emirates	35.20%	2006	5-17	17
Bahrain	36.30%	2009	5-8	6
Qatar	52.70%	2005	6-18	1
Kuwait	46.30%	2009	10-14	11
Iraq	7.30%	2005	7-13	16

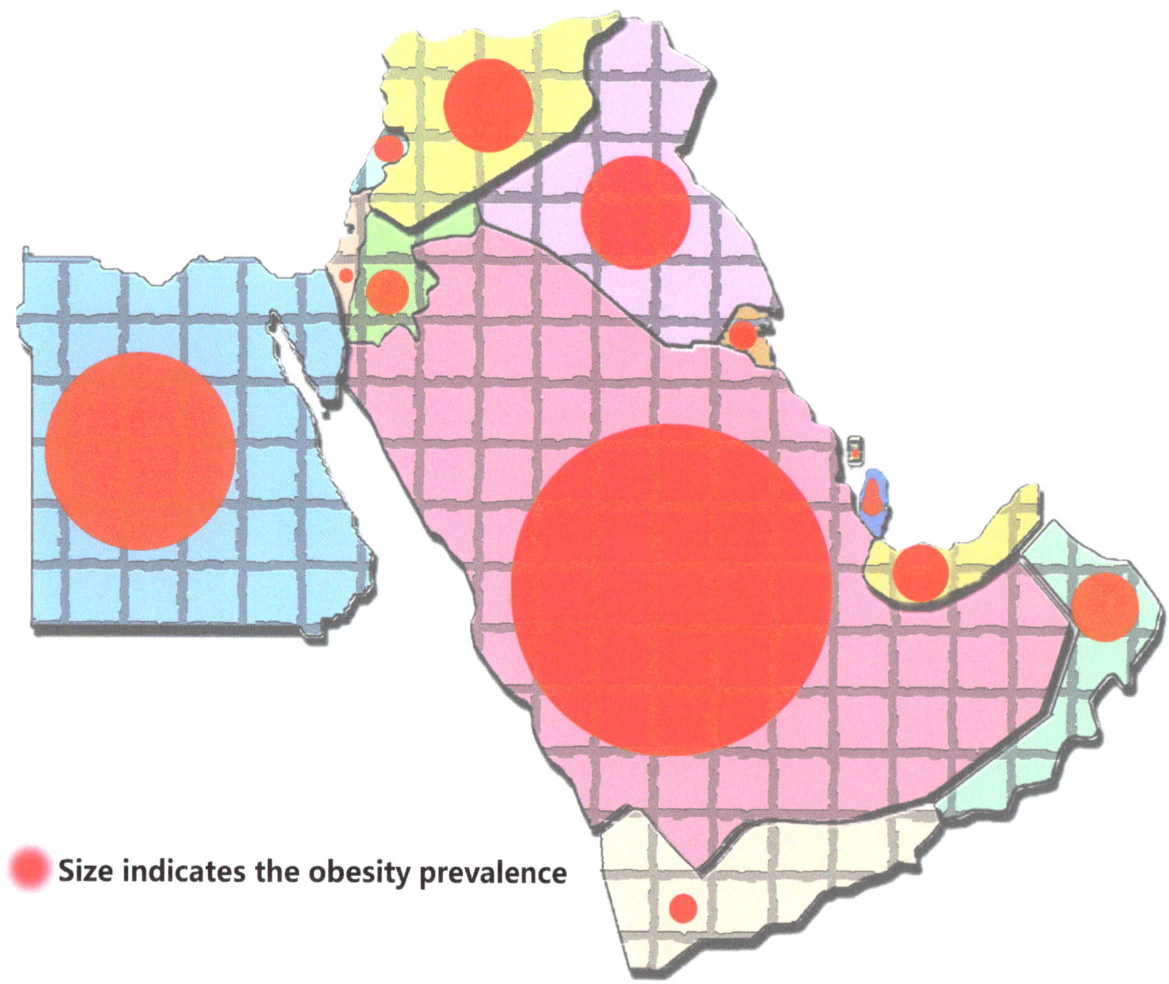

GRAINS

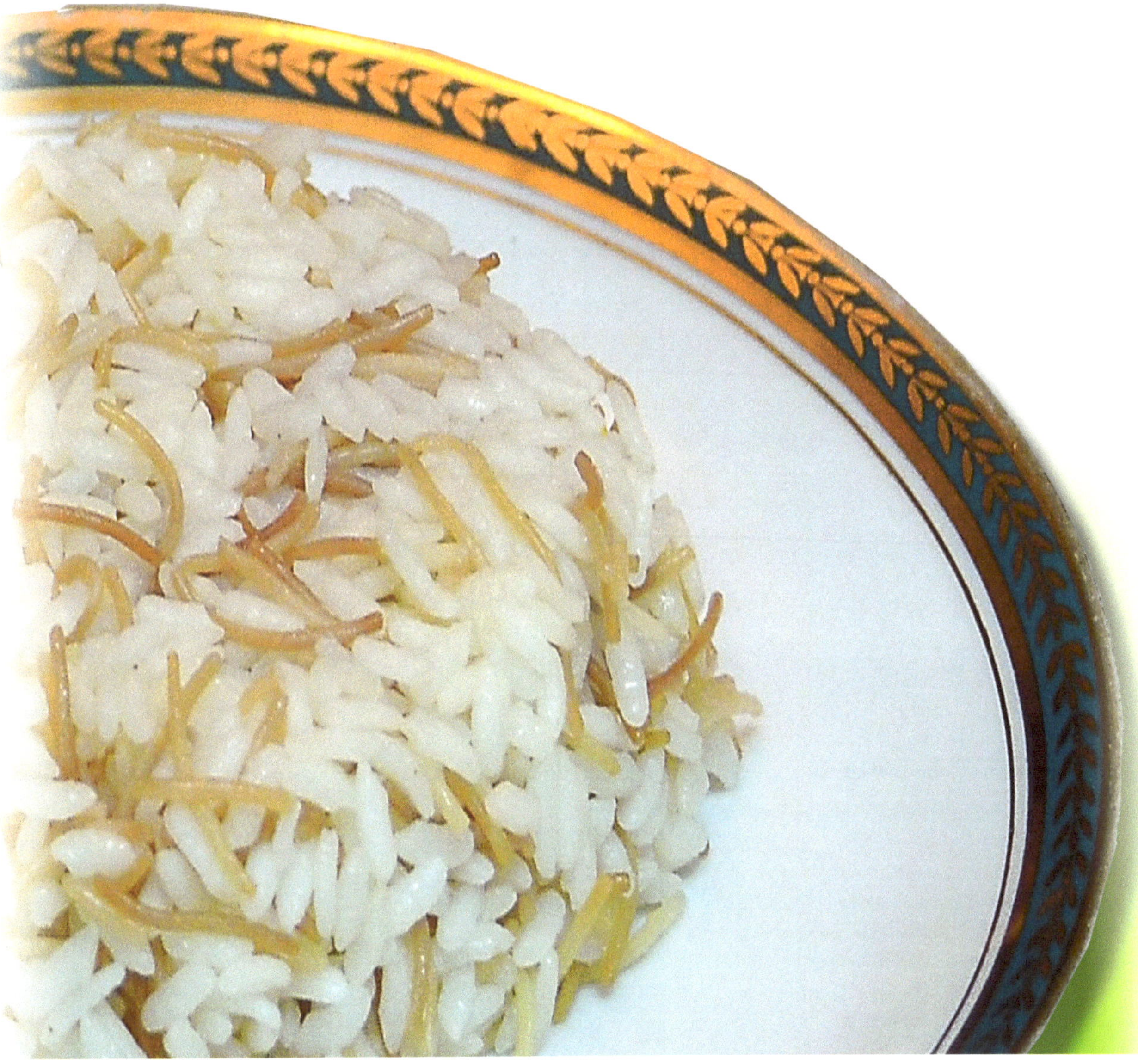

Bulgur Stewed with Fava Beans
(Burghul Bel Al-Foul)

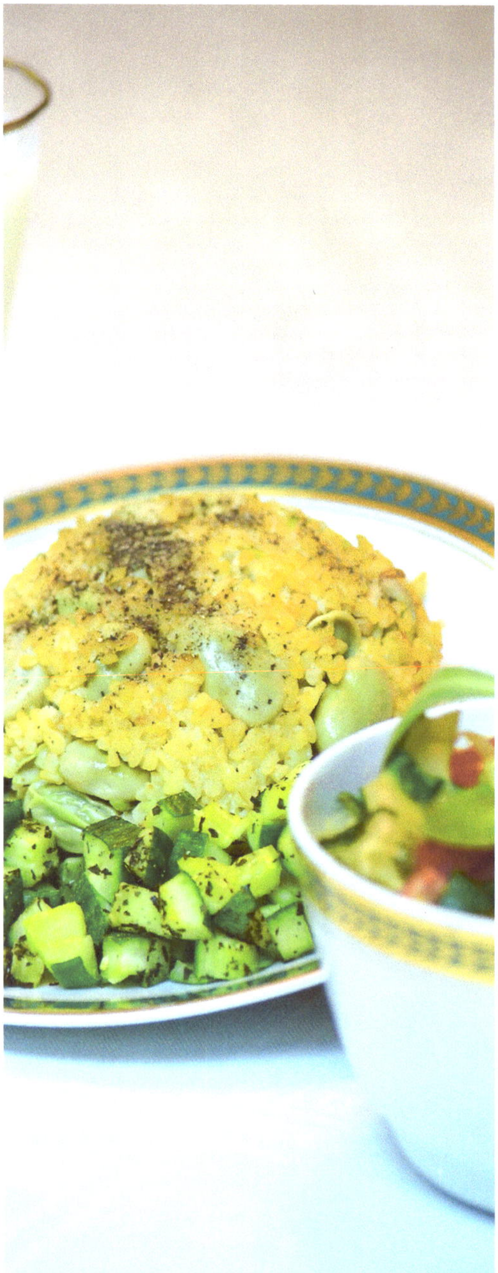

Traditional Recipe, 4 Servings, 4 Cups:

6 Tablespoons Corn Oil~81.464g
6 1/2 Tablespoons Chopped Onions~65.41g
1 1/2 cups Fresh Fava Beans~293.17g
3.5 oz. Ground Meat~98.84g
3/4 cup Bulgur Unenriched~161.73g
3 1/2 cups Water

Traditional Method of Preparation:

- Wash bulgur under running water; drain
- In a skillet, add beans with 1 1/2 cups of water and cook over medium heat for 10 minutes, until beans are tender
- In a cooking pan, heat oil and fry onions over medium-high heat for 5 minutes, until onions are light brown
- Combine meat with onions; continue cooking for 5 minutes, until meat is brown
- Drain beans and add bulgur to onions and meat with 2 cups of water; cover and cook over medium heat for 15 minutes
- Turn stove off; set for 5 minutes
- Ready to serve

Healthy Recipe, 4 Servings, 4 Cups:

5 teaspoons Olive Oil~22.45g
1/3 cup Chopped Onions~54.49g
1 1/4 cups Fresh Fava Beans~244.23g
3 oz. Lean Meat~82.3g
2/3 cup Bulgur Unenriched~134.73g
4 cups Water

Healthy Method of Preparation:

- Soak bulgur in 1 cup of warm water for 20 minutes, until water is absorbed
- Trim fat from steak and season with black pepper
- Place steak in a preheated nonstick skillet over medium-high heat for 8-10 minutes
- In a cooking pan, add fava beans with 1 cup of water and cook over medium heat for 5 minutes
- Add soaked bulgur with 1 cup of warm water and increase heat and cook over high heat for 10 minutes
- In a saucepan, add onions with 1 cup of water and bring to a boil over medium heat for 10 minutes. Add olive oil and reduce to low heat; stir frequently for 30 seconds
- Add sautéed onions to bulgur; stir twice
- Ready to serve

Nutritional Goal

Soaking bulgur in warm water for 20-30 minutes leads to a larger volume of yield, when less amount of bulgur is used. The proportion of bulgur to fava beans is 2:1 in the traditional recipe when it is 1.8:1 in the healthy recipe. After cooking, a cup of the traditional recipe weighs 244g, and a cup of the healthy one weighs 206g. This change results in calorie reduction of more than 5% in the healthy recipe when compared to the traditional recipe. This reduction of calories is related to reduction of carbohydrate, the bulgur. Steaming onions and beans instead of frying them, and adding olive oil to onions at the end, leads to saving of more than 15g of unnecessary fat, more than 30% reduction in calorie content, a much pleasurable taste, and high quality olive oil. The larger bulgur particles make a cup of the healthy recipe richer with fava bean. This makes the healthy recipe contain higher amounts of fiber, folic acid, potassium, and zinc. The healthy recipe is recommended to individuals with constipation and folate-deficiency anemia.

Nutrient Content	Traditional Recipe	Healthy Recipe
Portion	1 cup	1 cup
Weight (g)	244	206
Kilocalories (kcal)	428.41	246.99
Protein (g)	13.75	12
Carbohydrate (g)	40.7	33.69
Fat (g)	24.94	8.6
Saturated Fat (g)	4.21	1.6
Monounsaturated Fat (g)	6.59	5.5
Polyunsaturated Fat (g)	12.46	1.1
Trans Fatty Acid (g)	0.29	0.1
Cholesterol (g)	16.7	14.9
Omega-6 Linoleic (g)	11.92	0.65
Omega-3 Linolenic (g)	0.3	0.15
Fiber (g)	7.59	8.2
Sugar (g)	2.17	2.4
Water (L)	3.7	21.3
Thiamin (mg)	0.24	0.14
Riboflavin (mg)	0.17	0.11
Niacin (mg)	4.31	3.8
Vitamin B6 (mg)	0.27	0.35
Vitamin B12 (mcg)	0.533	0.54
Folate (DFE) mcg	15.4	28.6
Vitamin C (mg)	25.11	24.4
Vitamin D (mcg)	0	0
Vitamin A (RAE) (mcg)	77.44	0.1
Vitamin E (mg)	3.49	0.78
Calcium (mg)	37.39	33.9
Iron (mg)	2.9	2.16
Magnesium (mg)	99.7	94.23
Potassium (mg)	443.22	583
Zinc (mg)	2.32	2.6
Sodium (mg)	60	25.4

Portion 1 Cup

Number of Exchanges

Traditional Recipe
4 1/2 fat exchange (PUFA)
1 grain exchange
3/4 starch exchange
1 3/4 meat exchange (3/4 very lean,2/3 medium fat)

Healthy Recipe
1 1/4 fat exchange (MUFA)
1 grain exchange
2/3 starch exchange
1 1/4 meat exchange (2/3 very lean, 2/3 lean)

Calories from Macronutrients

Protein Carbohydrates Fat

Traditional Recipe

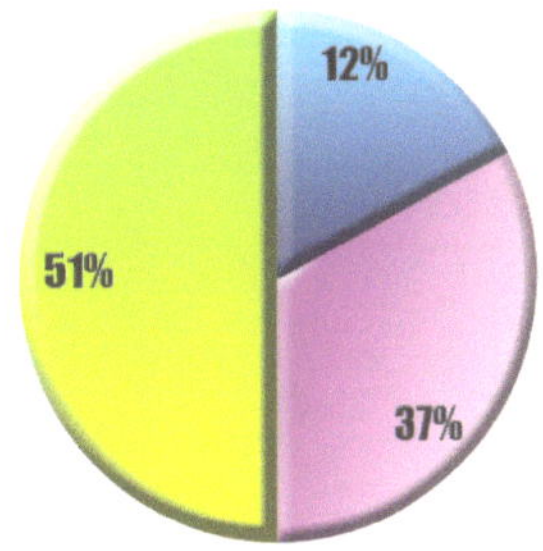

Healthy Recipe

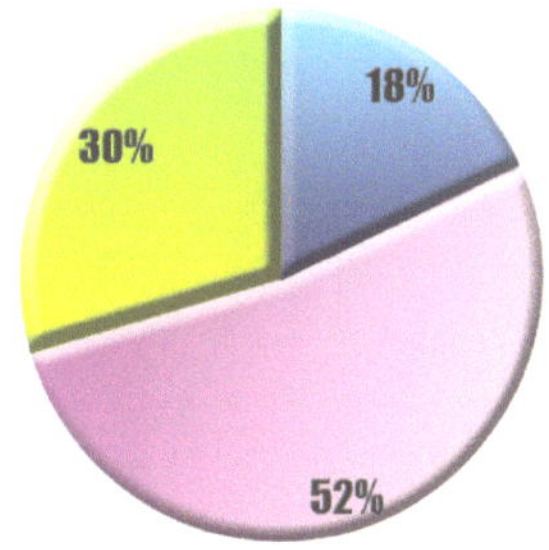

% Fiber Intake Compared to Average Daily Needs

Remaining Required Daily Consumed

Traditional Recipe

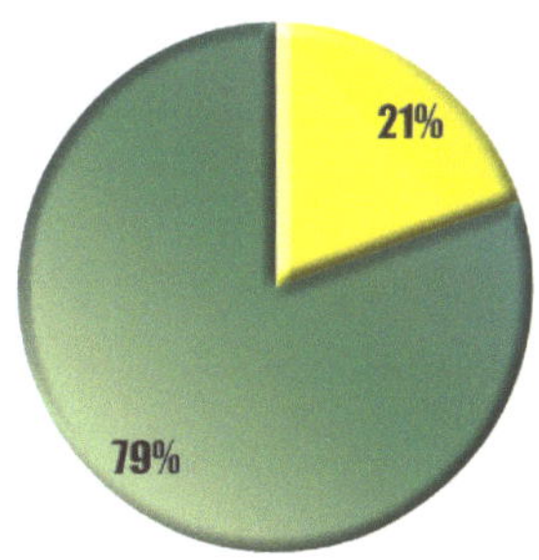

Healthy Recipe

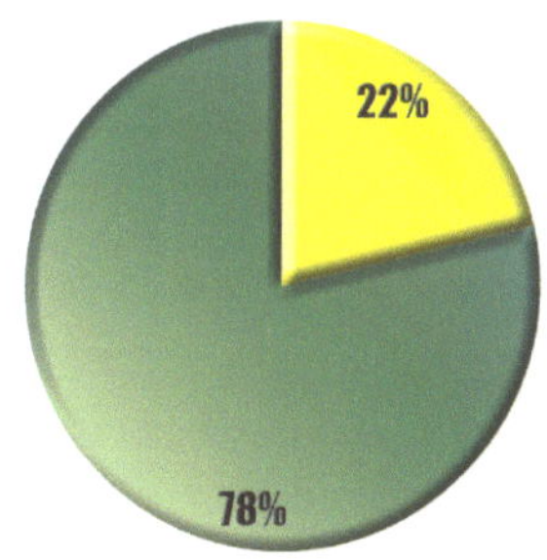

Recommended Portion Sizes & Meal Combinations

Traditional Recipe
(Calorie Controlled)

Men
1 1/3 cups of burghul bel al-foul
2 cups of cucumber salad
1 cup of regular yogurt

Women
3/4 cup of burghul bel al-foul
1cup of cucumber salad
2/3 cup of regular yogurt

Healthy Recipe
(Calorie Controlled & Content Balanced)

Men
2 cups of burghul bel al-foul
2 cups of cucumber salad
1 1/2 cups of lowfat yogurt

Women
1 1/3 cups of burghul bel al-foul
1cup of cucumber salad
2/3 cup of lowfat yogurt

Number of Exchanges in a Balanced Meal

Men
2 1/2 fat exchange (MUFA)
1 1/4 starch exchange
2 1/2 meat exchange (1 1/4 very lean, 1 1/4 lean)
1 2/3 grain exchange
2 1/2 milk exchange
2 non-starchy vegetable exchange

Women
1 2/3 fat exchange (MUFA)
1 starch exchange
1 3/4 meat exchange (1 very lean, 3/4 lean)
1 grain exchange
1 milk exchange

Bulgur Stewed with Tomatoes
(Burghul Be Al-Tamatum)

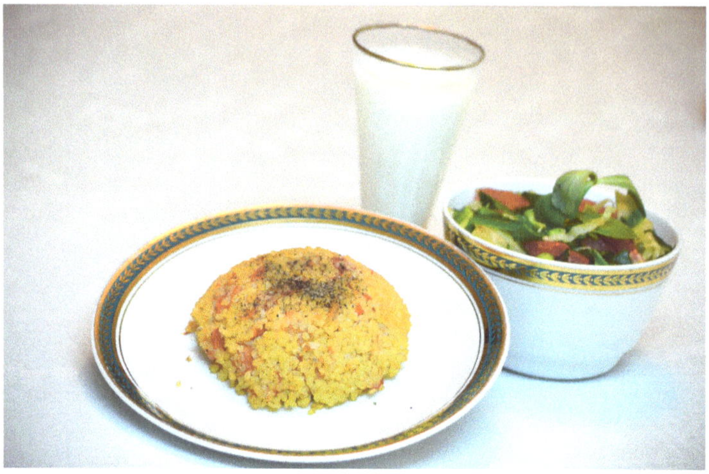

Traditional Recipe, 4 Servings, 4 Cups:

1 cup Bulgur~218.556g
1 2/3 cups Peeled Diced Tomatoes~395.082g
1/2 cup Chopped Onions~84g
3/4 cup Olive Oil~151g
2 cups Water

Traditional Method of Preparation:

- Wash bulgur under running water and drain
- In a cooking pan heat oil and fry onions over medium heat for 5 minutes until onions are lightly brown
- Combine tomatoes with onions and continue to cook for another 5 minutes
- Add bulgur with 2 cups of water; cover and cook over medium heat for 20 minutes
- Turn stove off; simmer for 5 minutes
- Ready to serve

Healthy Recipe, 4 Servings, 4 Cups:

3/4 cup Bulgur~155.116g
2 1/2 cups Peeled Diced Tomatoes~608.5g
1 cup Chopped Onions~178.98g
1 Tablespoon Olive Oil~13.4g
3 cups Water

Healthy Method of Preparation:

- Soak bulgur in 1 cup of warm water for 20 minutes until water is absorbed
- In a cooking pan, add tomatoes with 1 cup of water and cook over medium heat for 5 minutes
- Add soaked bulgur with 1 cup of warm water and continue to cook over medium heat for 20 minutes
- Turn stove off; cover and simmer for 5 minutes
- In a saucepan, add onions and 1 cup of water and bring to a boil over medium heat for 10 minutes
- Add olive oil and reduce heat to low, stir frequently for 30 seconds
- Add sautéed onions to cooked bulgur; stir twice
- Ready to serve

Nutritional Goal

The purpose of the modification is to reduce calories, to balance proportion of macronutrients, and to enrich food with nutrients. Comparing to the calorie content of the traditional recipe, calorie content of the healthy recipe is reduced by half. Fat is reduced by more than 80%; carbohydrate and protein are reduced by more than 10% in order to balance proportion of macronutrients in the healthy recipe. The healthy method of preparation preserves the quality of fat; it prevents the transition of fat into bad fat by heating the oil and reduces saturated fat by more than 80% in the healthy recipe. This cooking method also provides a larger volume of food; less amount of bulgur is used when compared to the traditional cooking method. This reduction of bulgur leads to reduction in fiber content in the healthy recipe, despite a greater amount of tomato and onions used. However, the nutritional analysis of the healthy recipe shows that it is enriched with more calcium, potassium, and folate, when compared to nutritional analysis of the traditional recipe. Therefore, the calorie content and nutritional values provided by the healthy recipe are more balanced when compared to the traditional recipe. The healthy recipe is highly recommended to individuals with high lipid profiles, heart disease, and excessive body weight.

Nutrient Content	Traditional Recipe	Healthy Recipe
Portion	1 cup	1 cup
Weight (g)	248	263.99
Kilocalories (kcal)	546.4	207.4
Protein (g)	7.75	6.5
Carbohydrate (g)	47.3	39.8
Fat (g)	38.8	4.2
Saturated Fat (g)	5.3	0.6
Monounsaturated Fat (g)	28	2.6
Polyunsaturated Fat (g)	4	0.8
Trans Fatty Acid (g)	0	0
Cholesterol (g)	0	0
Omega-6 Linoleic (g)	3.6	0.51
Omega-3 Linolenic (g)	0.32	0.04
Fiber (g)	11	9.5
Sugar (g)	3.7	6.1
Water (L)	5	3.7
Thiamin (mg)	0.2	0.2
Riboflavin (mg)	0.1	0.1
Niacin (mg)	3.4	2.9
Vitamin B6 (mg)	0.3	0.32
Vitamin B12 (mcg)	0	0
Folate (DFE) mcg	33.4	41.8
Vitamin C (mg)	13.8	22.2
Vitamin D (mcg)	0	0
Vitamin A (RAE) (mcg)	247	384.6
Vitamin E (mg)	4	0.93
Calcium (mg)	33.8	38.7
Iron (mg)	1.9	1.5
Magnesium (mg)	102	84.7
Potassium (mg)	485.7	584
Zinc (mg)	1.3	1.1
Sodium (mg)	16	15.6

Portion 1 Cup

Number of Exchanges

Traditional Recipe
1 1/3 grain exchange
1/2 non-starchy vegetable exchange
8 1/3 fat exchange (MUFA)

Healthy Recipe
1 grain exchange
1 non-starchy vegetable exchange
3/4 fat exchange (MUFA)

Calories from Macronutrients

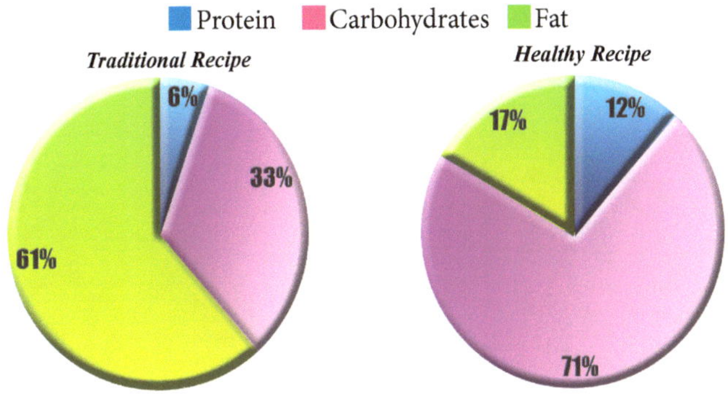

% Fiber Intake Compared to Average Daily Needs

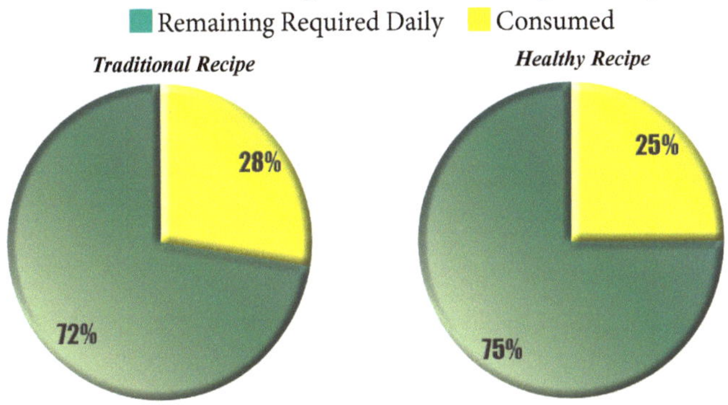

Recommended Portion Sizes & Meal Combinations

Traditional Recipe
(Calorie Controlled)

Men
1 1/4 cups of burghul be al-tamatum
1 1/4 cups of traditional green salad

Women
2/3 cup of burghul be al-tamatum
1 cup of traditional green salad

Healthy Recipe
(Calorie Controlled & Content Balanced)

Men
2 1/2 cups of burghul be al-tamatum
3 cups of green salad-drizzled with olive oil
1 cup of lowfat ayran

Women
1 1/2 cups of burghul be al-tamatum
1 1/2 cups of green salad-drizzled with olive oil
1 cup of lowfat ayran

Number of Exchanges in a Balanced Meal

Men
2 1/2 grain exchange
5 non-starchy vegetable exchange
5 fat exchange
1 milk exchange

Women
1 1/2 grain exchange
2 3/4 non-starchy vegetable exchange
2 1/2 fat exchange
1 milk exchange

Bulgur Stewed with Zucchini

(Burghul Be Al Kousa)

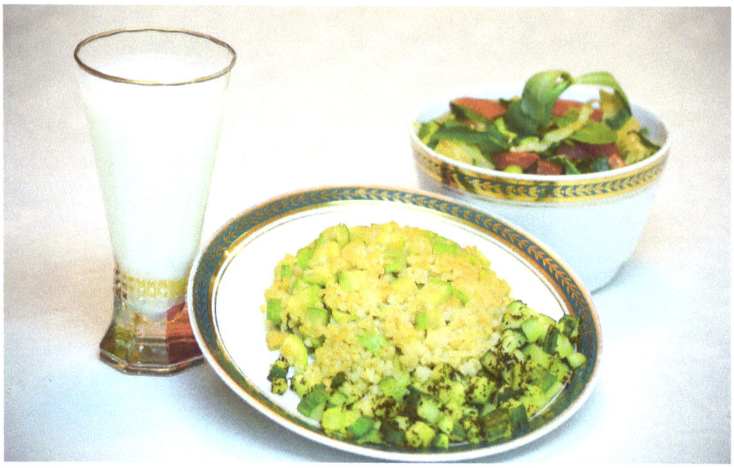

Traditional Recipe, 4 Servings, 4 Cups:

2/3 cup Chopped Onions~104g
1 1/4 cups Diced Zucchini~222g
5.5 oz. Ground Meat~156g
1 1/4 cups Bulgur Unenriched~255g
2/3 cup Corn Oil~128g
5 cups Water

Traditional Method of Preparation:

- Wash bulgur under running water; drain
- Heat corn oil in a pan and add onion to fry gently for 2 minutes, until onions are gold
- Season meat with black pepper and cook with onions for 10 minutes, until meat is brown; stir thoroughly
- Combine bulgur with meat and onions; stir twice
- Add 5 cups of water to pan; cover and cook for 30 minutes over medium heat
- Ready to serve

Healthy Recipe, 4 Servings, 4 Cups:

6 1/2 Tablespoons Chopped Onions~64g
1 1/2 cups Diced Zucchini~274g
3.5 oz. Lean Ground Meat~96g
3/4 cup Bulgur Unenriched~158g
2 Tablespoons Olive Oil~26g
6 cups Water

Healthy Method of Preparation:

- It is recommended not to wash packed bulgur to prevent nutrient loss. Soak bulgur in 1 cup of warm water until water is absorbed, for 20 minutes
- Season meat with black pepper and gently broil meat with 2 cup of water for 10 minutes until meat is brown
- Add zucchini with 1 cup of water to meat and stir for 2 minutes
- Combine soaked bulgur with zucchini and meat, stir over medium heat for 5 minutes
- Add 1 cup of warm water and cover for 20 minutes, until water evaporates
- Gently boil onion with 1 cup of water, until onions are thicker and water evaporates, about 10 minutes
- Add olive oil to onions and stir over low heat for 1 minute
- Turn off stove; add sautéed onions to cooked bulgur
- Ready to serve

Nutritional Goal

The purpose of modification is to reduce calorie content and to balance proportion of macronutrients. Although the two recipes provide a great variety of nutrients, the healthy recipe is more balanced and nutritious. The calorie content of the healthy recipe is reduced by more than 40% when compared to calorie content of the traditional recipe. Total fat, saturated fat, and trans fatty acid are reduced by more than half, when cholesterol is reduced by more than 15%. The healthy cooking method keeps a larger volume of food; it preserves the quality of fat and prevents the transition of good fat into bad fat. Fat calories are predominant in the traditional recipe; calories from macronutrients are well balanced in the healthy recipe. Thus, the healthy recipe is recommended to individuals with diabetes, excessive body weight, and high lipid profiles.

Nutrient Content	Traditional Recipe	Healthy Recipe
Portion	1 cup	1 cup
Weight (g)	228	206
Kilocalories (kcal)	478.5	246.98
Protein (g)	13.25	12
Carbohydrate (g)	41.55	33.68
Fat (g)	30.76	8.6
Saturated Fat (g)	5.17	1.6
Monounsaturated Fat (g)	8.24	5.47
Polyunsaturated Fat (g)	15.34	1.06
Trans Fatty Acid (g)	0.36	0.08
Cholesterol (g)	20.87	14.89
Omega-6 Linoleic (g)	14.8	0.65
Omega-3 Linolenic (g)	0.25	0.149
Fiber (g)	9.95	8.19
Sugar (g)	2.043	2.36
Water (L)	4.59	21.29
Thiamin (mg)	0.16	0.138
Riboflavin (mg)	0.13	0.113
Niacin (mg)	4.32	3.84
Vitamin B6 (mg)	0.37	0.35
Vitamin B12 (mcg)	0.66	0.54
Folate (DFE) mcg	28.03	28.6
Vitamin C (mg)	16.21	24.4
Vitamin D (mcg)	0	0
Vitamin A (RAE) (mcg)	0.124	0.097
Vitamin E (mg)	4.35	0.78
Calcium (mg)	35.9	33.97
Iron (mg)	2.26	2.16
Magnesium (mg)	104.4	94.23
Potassium (mg)	526.53	583.15
Zinc (mg)	2.74	2.6
Sodium (mg)	30.7	25.35

Portion 1 Cup

Number of Exchanges

Traditional Recipe
1/2 non-starchy vegetable exchange
1 1/4 meat exchange (medium fat)
1 2/3 grain exchange
7 fat exchange (PUFA)

Healthy Recipe
1/2 non-starchy vegetable exchange
3/4 meat exchange (lean)
1 grain exchange
1 1/3 fat exchange (MUFA)

Calories from Macronutrients

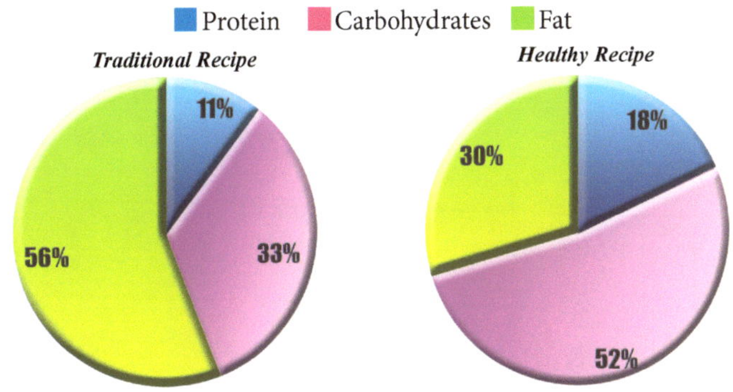

% Fiber Intake Compared to Average Daily Needs

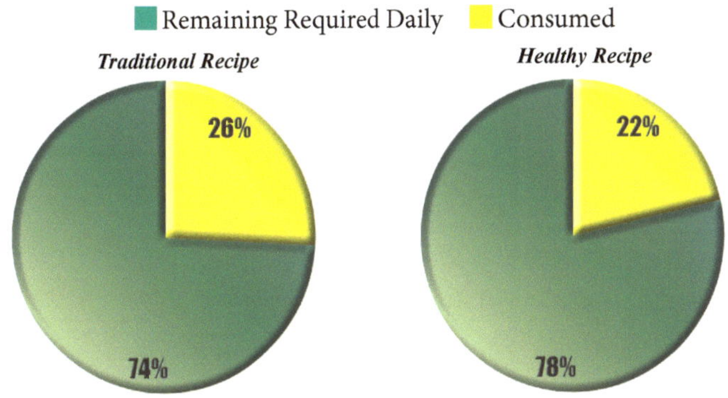

Recommended Portion Sizes & Meal Combinations

Traditional Recipe
(Calorie Controlled)

Men
1 1/2 cups of bulghur be al kousa
2 cups of cucumber salad

Women
1 cup of bulghur be al kousa
1/2 cup of cucumber salad

Healthy Recipe
(Calorie Controlled & Content Balanced)

Men
2 1/4 cups of bulghur be al kousa
4 cups of cucumber salad
1 cup of lowfat ayran

Women
1 1/3 cups of bulghur be al kousa
2 cups of cucumber salad
1 cup of lowfat ayran

Number of Exchanges in a Balanced Meal

Men
5 non-starchy vegetable exchange
1 2/3 meat exchange (lean)
2 1/4 grain exchange
3 fat exchange (MUFA)
1 milk exchange

Women
2 2/3 non-starchy vegetable exchange
1 meat exchange (lean)
1 1/3 grain exchange
1 3/4 fat exchange (MUFA)
1 milk exchange

Cracked Wheat with Meat

(Jaresh Madroub)

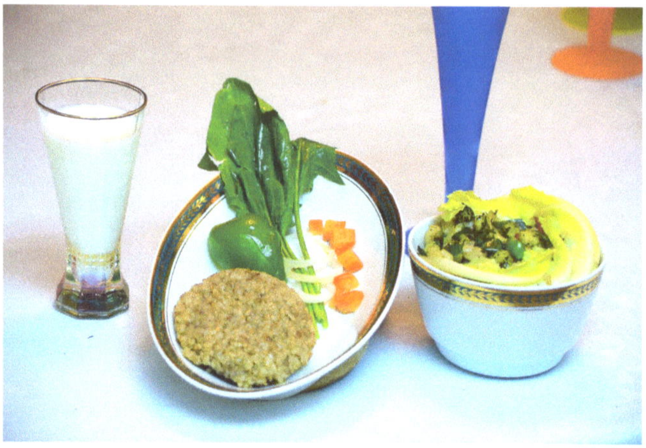

Traditional Recipe, 4 Servings, 4 Cups:

1 cup Diced Tomatoes~264.55g
1 cup Ground Wheat~224.85g
3 Tablespoons Chopped Onions~29.34g
7 oz. Medium Fat Meat~197g
1 1/4 teaspoons Black Pepper~2 1/2g
6 1/2 Tablespoons Corn Oil~88.146g
9 Cups Water

Traditional Method of Preparation:

- Wash wheat under running water until water is clear
- In a cooking pan, heat oil and fry onions over moderate heat for 5 minutes, until onions are golden brown
- Season meat with black pepper and place it with onions, cook over medium heat for 10 minutes; stir frequently to prevent sticking
- Add tomatoes, wheat, and water into mixture; enough water to cover food
- Cover and cook over moderate heat for 40 minutes
- Reduce heat, and continue cooking over low heat for 5 minutes, until water evaporates
- Crack food using mortar
- Ready to serve

Healthy Recipe, 4 Servings, 4 Cups:

1 3/4 cups Diced Tomatoes~448.404g
3/4 cup Ground Wheat~169.85g
3/4 cup Chopped Onions~135.88g
2.4 oz. Lean Meat~68g
3 teaspoons Black Pepper~6g
4 1/2 Tablespoons Ground Flaxseed~33.97g
5 Cups Water

Healthy Method of Preparation:

- Soak wheat in hot water for 20 minutes until water is absorbed
- In a cooking pan combine meat, black pepper, and 1 cup of water, cook over moderate heat for 10 minutes
- Add onions and 1 cup of water to meat, cover and cook for 10 minutes
- Combine tomatoes, wheat, 3 cups of water with meat and onions,
  cover and cook over moderate heat for another 30 minutes
- Sprinkle food with ground flaxseed before cracking it
- Crack food using mortar
- Ready to serve

Nutritional Goal

The purpose of modification is to reduce calories, to balance macronutrients proportion, and to enrich food with fiber and nutrients. A comparison between the traditional and the healthy recipes shows that the healthy recipe has multiple health benefits. The calorie content of the healthy recipe is reduced by more than half when compared to calorie content of the traditional recipe. The proportion of macronutrients is well balanced in the healthy recipe since fat calories are replaced with carbohydrates and protein calories. Total fat, saturated fat, and trans fatty acid are reduced by more than 70% and cholesterol is reduced by more than half as well. The nutritional analysis shows that the healthy recipe is enriched with fiber, folate, and calcium when compared to their levels in the traditional recipe. The calorie content, proportion of macronutrients, and nutrient enrichments are factors to recommend the healthy recipe to individuals with diabetes, constipation, osteoporosis, high lipid profiles, and excessive body weight.

Nutrient Content	Traditional Recipe	Healthy Recipe
Portion	1 cup	1 cup
Weight (g)	240	247.9
Kilocalories (kcal)	533.63	254
Protein (g)	17.3	11.6
Carbohydrate (g)	51	43.3
Fat (g)	31.3	5.9
Saturated Fat (g)	6.2	1
Monounsaturated Fat (g)	9.9	1.4
Polyunsaturated Fat (g)	12.9	3
Trans Fatty Acid (g)	0.5	0.1
Cholesterol (g)	33.5	10.5
Omega-6 Linoleic (g)	0.3	0.2
Omega-3 Linolenic (g)	0.33	2
Fiber (g)	7.5	8.7
Sugar (g)	2.1	4.7
Water (L)	5	4.3
Thiamin (mg)	0.2	0.3
Riboflavin (mg)	0.3	0.2
Niacin (mg)	5.9	4.1
Vitamin B6 (mg)	0.5	0.4
Vitamin B12 (mcg)	1.1	0.4
Folate (DFE) mcg	40	49.2
Vitamin C (mg)	9.4	16.8
Vitamin D (mcg)	0	0
Vitamin A (RAE) (mcg)	168.5	283.6
Vitamin E (mg)	4	0.88
Calcium (mg)	37	56.7
Iron (mg)	3.5	2.8
Magnesium (mg)	157	150
Potassium (mg)	541.2	600
Zinc (mg)	3.8	2.5
Sodium (mg)	44	26

Portion 1 Cup

Number of Exchanges

Traditional Recipe
1 1/3 grain exchange
1 2/3 meat exchange (medium fat)
5 fat exchange (PUFA)
1/3 non-starchy vegetable exchange

Healthy Recipe
1 grain exchange
2/3 meat exchange (lean)
3 1/3 fat exchange (Omega-3-FA)
2/3 non-starchy vegetable exchange

Calories from Macronutrients

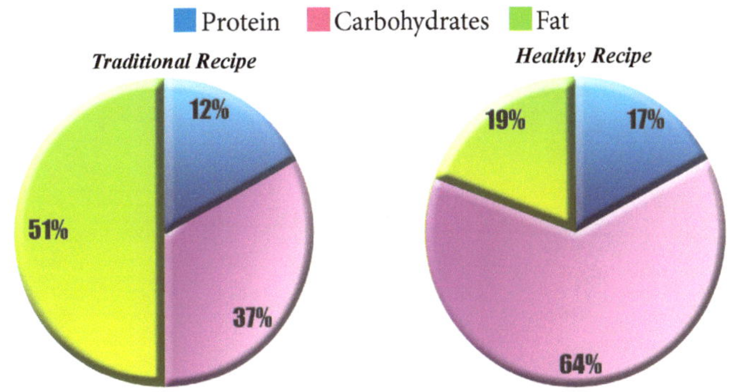

% Fiber Intake Compared to Average Daily Needs

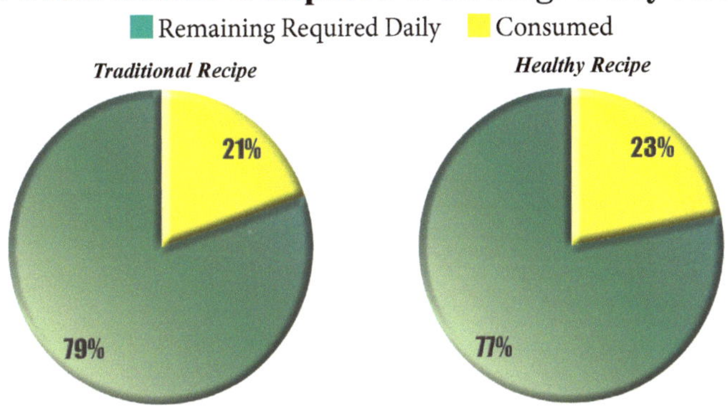

Recommended Portion Sizes & Meal Combinations

Traditional Recipe
(Calorie Controlled)

Men
1 1/4 cup of jaresh madroub
2 cups of green salad-drizzled with vinegar & olive oil

Women
3/4 cup of jaresh madroub
2 cups of green salad-drizzled with vinegar & olive oil

Healthy Recipe
(Calorie Controlled & Content Balanced)

Men
2 1/4 cups jaresh madroub
3 cups of green salad-drizzled with vinegar
1 cup of lowfat ayran

Women
1 1/2 cups of jaresh madroub
1 cup of green salad-drizzled with vinegar
1 cup of lowfat ayran

Number of Exchanges in a Balanced Meal

Men
2 1/4 grain exchange
1 1/3 meat exchange (lean)
7 2/3 fat exchange (Omega-3-FA)
4 1/2 non-starchy vegetable exchange
1 milk exchange

Women
1 1/2 grain exchange
1 meat exchange (lean)
5 fat exchange (Omega-3-FA)
2 non-starchy vegetable exchange
1 milk exchange

Groat Grain
(Farekah)

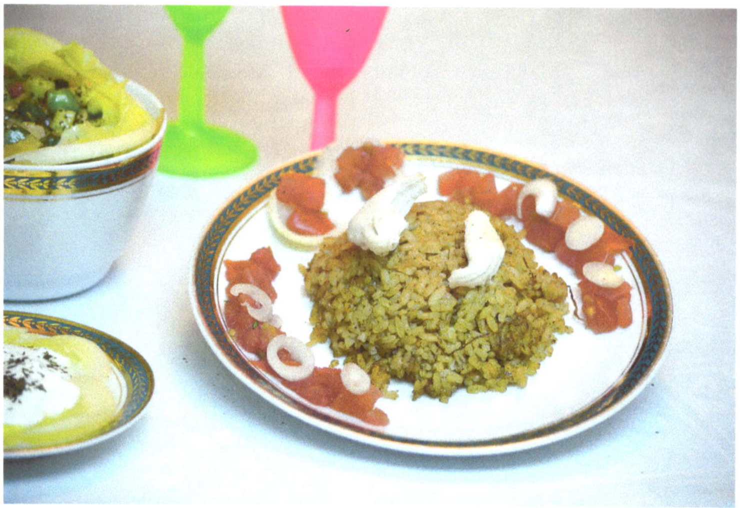

Traditional Recipe, 4 Servings, 4 Cups:

1 2/3 cups Groat Wheat~260g
3/4 cup Chopped Onions~130g
1/2 cup Corn Oil~117g
5 cups Water

Healthy Recipe, 4 Servings, 4 Cups:

1 1/2 cups Groat Wheat~224g
1 1/2 cups Chopped Onions~224g
2 1/2 teaspoons Canola Oil~11.2g
1 1/2 Tablespoons Ground Flaxseed~11.2g
5 cups Water

Traditional Method of Preparation:

- Wash groat under running water, until water is clear
- In a cooking pan, heat oil and fry onions over medium heat for 5 minutes, until they are brown
- Combine groat with onions, continue frying for 5 minutes; stir frequently
- Add water, and cook over medium heat for 40 minutes
- Reduce heat, cover and continue to cook over low heat for 5 minutes until water evaporates
- Ready to serve

Healthy Method of Preparation:

- Soak groat in warm water for 20 minutes, until water is absorbed
- In a cooking pan, bring 5 cups of water to boil, add onions and groat; and cook over medium heat for 40 minutes
- Reduce heat, add canola oil, cover and cook over low heat for 3 minutes
- Add flaxseed, stir twice
- Ready to serve

Nutritional Goal

The purpose of modification is to reduce calorie content, to improve fat quality, and to add nutritional value to food. Calorie content of the healthy recipe is reduced by more than half when compared to calorie content of the traditional recipe. In the healthy recipe, total fat, saturated fat, and omega-6-FA are reduced by more than 75%, when Omega-3-FA is increased by more than 200%. The measurable change in fat content leads to well balance macronutrients in the healthy recipe, when compared to the traditional recipe. The nutritional analysis of the healthy recipe demonstrates greater levels of fiber, folate, vitamin C, and vitamin A, when compared to the nutritional analysis of the traditional recipe. The healthy recipe is recommended to individuals with high lipid profiles, excessive body weight, and folate deficiency anemia.

Nutrient Content	Traditional Recipe	Healthy Recipe
Portion	1 cup	1 cup
Weight (g)	208	224
Kilocalories (kcal)	696.32	276.6
Protein (g)	38.5	10.9
Carbohydrate (g)	52.4	48.6
Fat (g)	38.6	6.2
Saturated Fat (g)	7.3	1
Monounsaturated Fat (g)	10.4	2.6
Polyunsaturated Fat (g)	19	2
Trans Fatty Acid (g)	0.1	0.01
Cholesterol (g)	0	0
Omega-6 Linoleic (g)	18	0.5
Omega-3 Linolenic (g)	0.26	1.2
Fiber (g)	7	7.3
Sugar (g)	1.4	2.5
Water (L)	8	5
Thiamin (mg)	0.22	0.2
Riboflavin (mg)	0.74	0.23
Niacin (mg)	24.3	5.3
Vitamin B6 (mg)	0.54	0.3
Vitamin B12 (mcg)	1.9	0.2
Folate (DFE) mcg	33	36.5
Vitamin C (mg)	2.1	3.6
Vitamin D (mcg)	0	0
Vitamin A (RAE) (mcg)	0.2	0.34
Vitamin E (mg)	6	1.2
Calcium (mg)	179.5	46
Iron (mg)	6.2	2.1
Magnesium (mg)	198	145.8
Potassium (mg)	1705	437.4
Zinc (mg)	1.6	1.6
Sodium (mg)	8781	947.9

Portion 1 Cup

Number of Exchanges

Traditional Recipe
2 1/4 grain exchange
6 1/2 fat exchange (PUFA)

Healthy Recipe
2 grain exchange
1 2/3 fat exchange (2/3 MUFA,
1 Omega-3-FA)
1/3 non-starchy vegetable exchange

Calories from Macronutrients

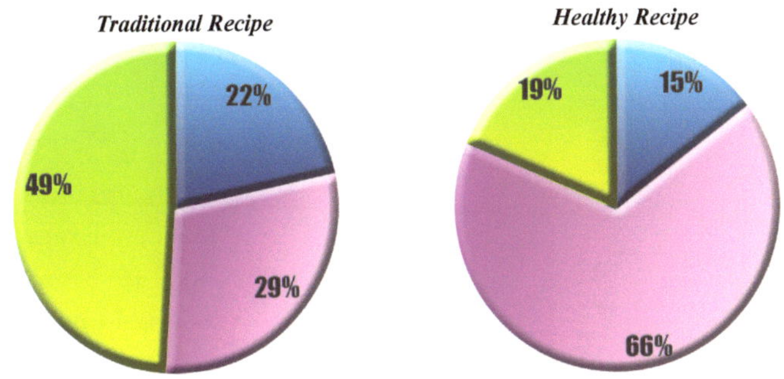

% Fiber Intake Compared to Average Daily Needs

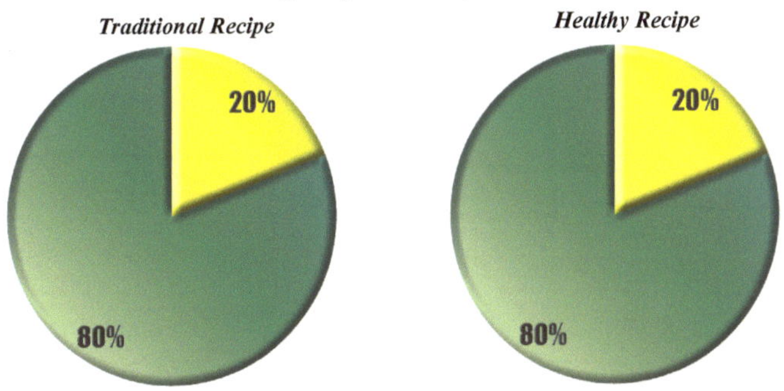

Recommended Portion Sizes & Meal Combinations

Traditional Recipe
(Calorie Controlled)

Men
3/4 cup of farekah
1 serving of boiled/grilled chicken breast(3oz)
3/4 cup of regular plain yogurt

Women
1/2 cup of farekah
1/3 serving of boiled/grilled chicken breast(1oz)
1/2 cup of regular plain yogurt

Healthy Recipe
(Calorie Controlled & Content Balanced)

Men
1 2/3 cups of farekah
1 serving of boiled/grilled chicken breast (3oz)
2 cups of green salad-drizzled with vinegar
2/3 cup of lowfat plain yogurt

Women
1 cup of farekah
2/3 serving of boiled/grilled chicken breast (2oz)
1 1/2 cups of green salad-drizzled with vinegar
1/2 cup of lowfat plain yogurt

Number of Exchanges in a Balanced Meal

Men
3 1/4 grains exchange
2 2/3 non-starchy vegetable exchange
3 fat exchange (1 MUFA,
2 Omega-3-FA)
3 meat exchange (lean)
1 milk exchange

Women
2 grain exchange
2 non-starchy vegetable exchange
1 2/3 fat exchange (2/3 MUFA,
1 Omega-3-FA)
2 meat exchange (lean)
1 milk exchange

Lentils with Bulgur Wheat
(Mujadara)

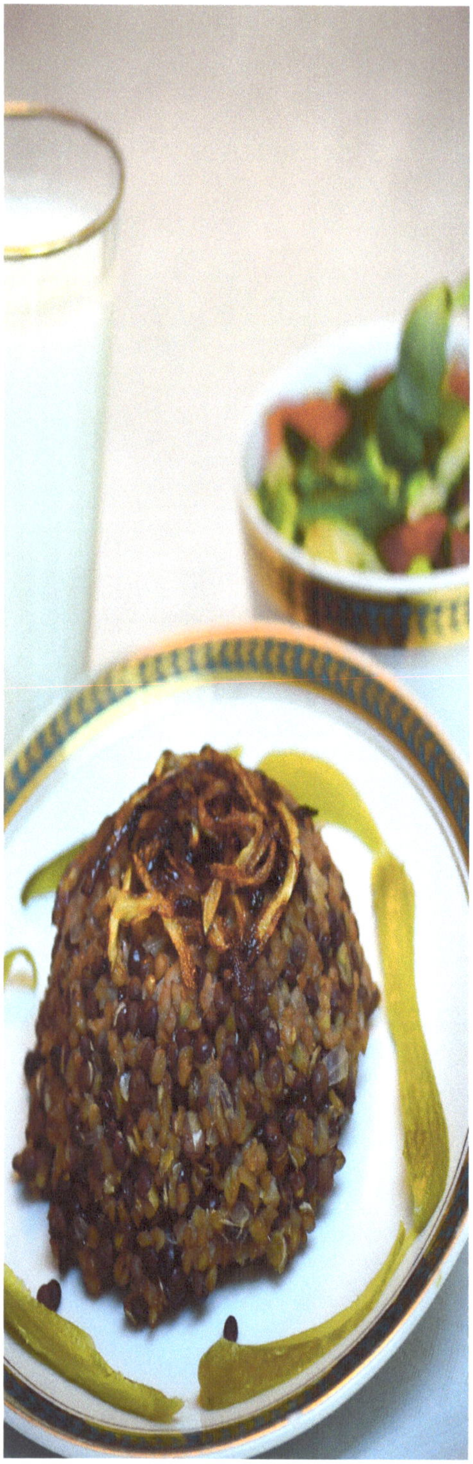

Traditional Recipe, 4 Servings, 4 Cups:

3 3/4 teaspoons Olive Oil~17.28g
3/4 cup Chopped Onions~135.36g
1/4 cup Shredded Onions~40g
6 1/2 Tablespoons Bulgur~83.2g
3/4 cup Brown Lentils~151.04g
2 1/2 teaspoons Corn Oil~11.67g
8 cups Water

Traditional Method of Preparation:

- Wash and drain lentils and bulgur separately
- In a cooking pan, heat oil and fry onions over medium heat for 3 minutes, until onions are brown
- Add bulgur and continue frying for 1 minute; stir continuously. Combine lentils with onions and bulgur and cook for another 3 minutes
- Add 8 cups of water to pan and bring it to gentle boil. Cover and cook over medium heat for another 25 minutes
- In a separate saucepan, heat olive oil and fry shredded Onions over medium heat for 4 minutes.; stir frequently to prevent sticking
- Optional: Top or mix the fried shredded onions with ready-to-serve Mujadara

Healthy Recipe, 4 Servings, 4 Cups:

1 Tablespoon Olive Oil~13.5g
1/2 cup Chopped Onions~75.5g
1/3 cup Shredded Onions~52.5g
5 Tablespoons Bulgur~64g
2/3 cup Brown Lentils~128.5g
7 cups Water

Healthy Method of Preparation:

- It is recommended not to wash packed lentils and bulgur to prevent nutrient loss. Soak bulgur and lentils, each separately in 1 cup of warm water for 20 minutes, until water is absorbed
- In a cooking pan, bring 4 1/2 cups of water to boil and combine chopped onions, soaked bulgur and lentils. Cover and cook over medium heat for 20 minutes, until water evaporates.
- In a saucepan, place shredded onions with 1/2 cup of water and bring to a boil over medium heat for 10 minutes.
- Add 1 tablespoon of olive oil and reduce to low heat; stir frequently for 30 seconds
- Optional: Top or mix the pan-fried onions with ready-to-serve Mujadara

Nutritional Goal

The modification aims to reduce calorie content, improve quality of fat, and reduce sodium content of food. The total calories of the healthy recipe are reduced by more than 25% when compared to the total calories of the traditional recipe. The quantity and quality of fat are controlled since the healthy recipe is trans fatty acid free and contains less than 52% total fat and less than 50% saturated fat. The Sodium content is also reduced by more than 15% in the healthy recipe when compared to the sodium content of the traditional recipe. The healthy recipe is recommended to individuals with excessive body weight, high lipid profiles, and high blood pressure.

Nutrient Content	Traditional Recipe	Healthy Recipe
Portion	1 cup	1 cup
Weight (g)	222.72	231.75
Kilocalories (kcal)	286.665	212.43
Protein (g)	12.7	10.56
Carbohydrate (g)	43	34.9
Fat (g)	8	3.9
Saturated Fat (g)	1.1	0.55
Monounsaturated Fat (g)	4	2.59
Polyunsaturated Fat (g)	2.5	0.6
Trans Fatty Acid (g)	0.008	0
Cholesterol (g)	0	0
Omega-6 Linoleic (g)	2.12	0.35
Omega-3 Linolenic (g)	0.06	0.03
Fiber (g)	15.9	13.2
Sugar (g)	2.73	2.09
Water (L)	5.85	4.8
Thiamin (mg)	0.39	0.33
Riboflavin (mg)	0.115	0.09
Niacin (mg)	2.08	1.69
Vitamin B6 (mg)	0.34	0.28
Vitamin B12 (mcg)	0	0
Folate (DFE) mcg	194.8	164.5
Vitamin C (mg)	4.46	3.47
Vitamin D (mcg)	0	0
Vitamin A (RAE) (mcg)	1.02	0.84
Vitamin E (mg)	1.22	0.58
Calcium (mg)	38.136	30.8
Iron (mg)	3.47	2.9
Magnesium (mg)	84.57	69.1
Potassium (mg)	509.1	420.12
Zinc (mg)	2.3	1.9
Sodium (mg)	7.2	5.75

Portion 1 Cup

Number of Exchanges

Traditional Recipe
1 2/3 fat exchange (1MUFA, 2/3PUFA)
1/3 starch exchange
1/3 meat exchange (very lean)
1/2 grain exchange
1/4 non-starchy vegetable exchange

Healthy Recipe
3/4 fat exchange (MUFA)
1 starch exchange
1 meat exchange (very lean)
1/3 grain exchange
1/4 non-starchy vegetable exchange

Calories from Macronutrients

Protein | Carbohydrates | Fat

Traditional Recipe

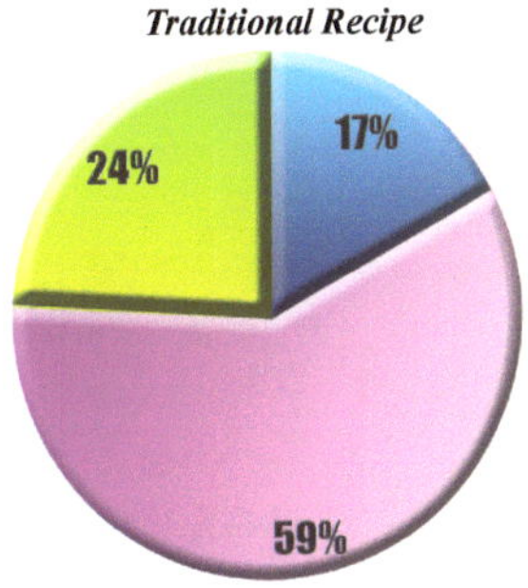

Healthy Recipe

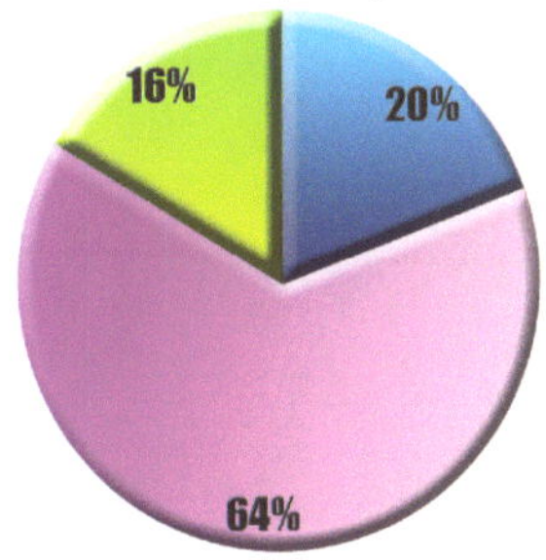

% Fiber Intake Compared to Average Daily Needs

Remaining Required Daily | Consumed

Traditional Recipe

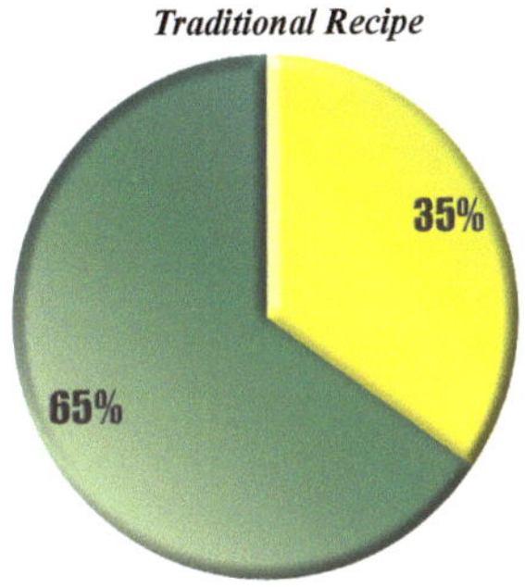

Healthy Recipe

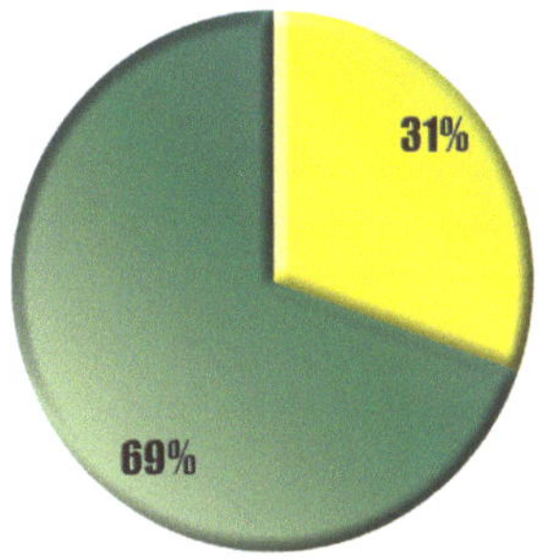

Recommended Portion Sizes & Meal Combinations

Traditional Recipe
(Calorie Controlled)

Men
1 3/4 cups of Mujadara
1/2 cup of pickled cucumber & beets
1 cup of green salad
1 cup of regular plain yogurt

Women
1 cup of Mujadara
1/2 cup of pickled cucumber & beets
1 cup of green salad
1/2 cup of regular plain yogurt

Healthy Recipe
(Calorie Controlled & Content Balanced)

Men
2 1/3 cups of Mujadara
1/2 cup of pickled cucumber & beets
1 cup of green salad-drizzled with olive oil
1 cup lowfat plain yogurt

Women
1 1/4 cups of Mujadara
1/2 cup of pickled cucumber & beets
1 cup of green salad-drizzled with olive oil
2/3 cup lowfat plain yogurt

Number of Exchanges in a Balanced Meal

Men
2 3/4 fat exchange (MUFA)
1 2/3 non-starchy vegetable exchange
1 grain exchange
3/4 starch exchange
3/4 meat exchange (very lean)
1 1/2 milk exchange

Women
2 fat exchange (MUFA)
1/4 non-starchy vegetable exchange
1/2 grain exchange
1/3 starch exchange
1/3 meat exchange (very lean)
1 milk exchange

Lentils Stewed with Rice
(Moa'adas)

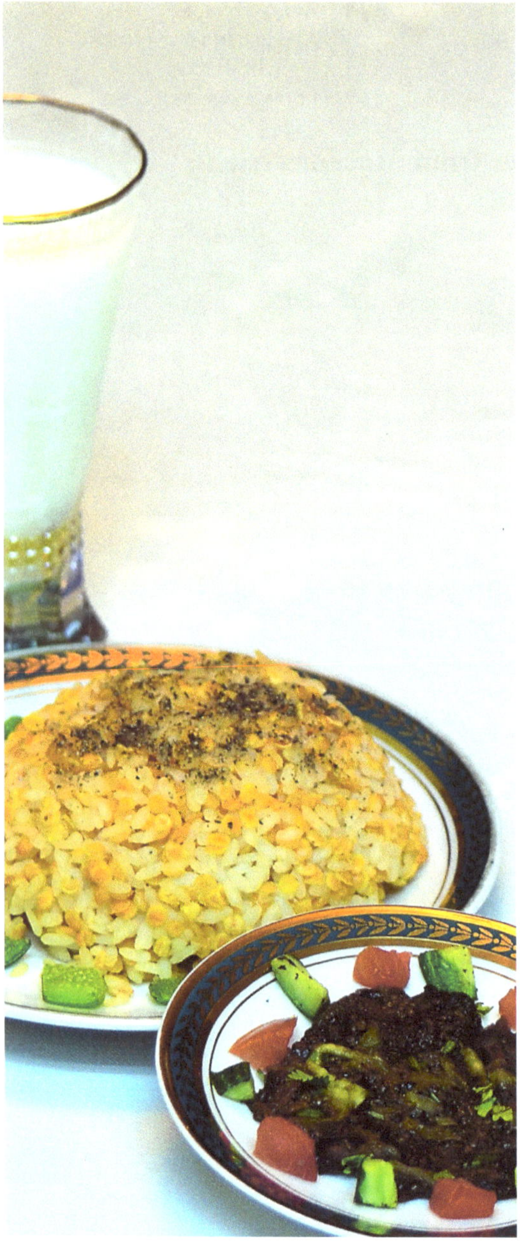

Traditional Recipe, 4 Servings, 4 Cups:

3/4 cup Rice Unenriched~168g
1/4 cup Pink Lentils~52g
1 1/2 Tablespoons Olive Oil~20g (corn oil maybe used)
1/3 cup Chopped Onions~62.4g
2 2/3 Tablespoons Corn Oil~36g
2 1/2 cups Water

Traditional Method of Preparation:

- Wash and drain rice; soak rice in cold water for 10 minutes
- In a saucepan, heat olive oil and fry onions over medium heat for 5 minutes, until onions are golden brown
- Remove half of fried onions and keep aside
- In a cooking pan, heat corn oil and stir rice and lentils for 2 minutes
- Combine half of fried onions and 2 1/2 cups of water with rice and lentils
- Cook over medium heat for 20 minutes
- Reduce heat, cover and cook over low heat for 5 minutes
- Place food in a serving plate, garnish with sautéed onions
- Ready to serve

Healthy Recipe, 4 Servings, 4 Cups:

3/4 cup Rice Unenriched~152.28g
3/4 cup Red Lentils~141g
1 1/2 teaspoons Olive Oil~6.3g
3/4 cup Chopped Onions~112.8g
3/4 cup Shredded Onions~112.8g
5 2/3 teaspoons Ground Flaxseed~14g
3 1/2 cups Water

Healthy Method of Preparation:

- Wash rice under running water; soak in warm water for 20 minutes
- In a cooking pan, combine rice, lentils, chopped onions and 3 cups of water; cover and cook over medium heat for 25 minutes
- Reduce heat, add flaxseed and continue cooking over low heat for another 5 minutes
- In a saucepan, place shredded onions with 1/2 cup of water and bring to boil over medium heat for 5 minutes, until onions are golden and thicker and water evaporates
- Add olive oil and reduce to low heat; stir frequently for 30 seconds
- Place food in serving plate, garnish with sautéed onions
- Ready to serve

Nutritional Goal

The healthy recipe is nutritionally superior to the traditional recipe. The change of rice:lentil ratio adds numerous health benefits to food. The healthy recipe is enriched with plant-source protein and complex carbohydrate leading to a reduction in fat and calorie contents. Nutritional analysis shows that total calories of the healthy recipe is reduced by more than 20%, when total fat and saturated fat are reduced by more than 75%, when compared to the traditional recipe. Also, the ratio of omega-6: omega-3 is improved; the ratio of the traditional recipe is 48:1 when the ratio of the healthy recipe is 1:1. Most importantly, the fiber content of the healthy recipe is increased by more than 100%, when compared to the fiber content of the traditional recipe. Thiamin, riboflavin, vitamin B6, folate, vitamin A, calcium, magnesium, potassium, and zinc are richer in the healthy recipe, when compared to their levels in the traditional recipe. The healthy recipe is recommended to individuals with heart disease, high lipid profiles, malnutrition, osteoporosis, excessive body weight, and constipation.

Nutrient Content	Traditional Recipe	Healthy Recipe
Portion	1 cup	1 cup
Weight (g)	170	216
Kilocalories (kcal)	297.6	215.8
Protein (g)	4.3	6.8
Carbohydrate (g)	37.5	41.7
Fat (g)	14	2.4
Saturated Fat (g)	1.9	0.3
Monounsaturated Fat (g)	6	1.3
Polyunsaturated Fat (g)	6	0.7
Trans Fatty Acid (g)	0.02	0
Cholesterol (g)	0	0
Omega-6 Linoleic (g)	5.7	0.19
Omega-3 Linolenic (g)	0.12	0.32
Fiber (g)	2.9	6.2
Sugar (g)	0.9	3.2
Water (L)	5.6	4.8
Thiamin (mg)	0.3	0.29
Riboflavin (mg)	0.03	0.1
Niacin (mg)	1.8	1.8
Vitamin B6 (mg)	0.04	0.14
Vitamin B12 (mcg)	0	0
Folate (DFE) mcg	121	151.9
Vitamin C (mg)	1.2	4.2
Vitamin D (mcg)	0	0
Vitamin A (RAE) (mcg)	0.6	1.7
Vitamin E (mg)	2.1	0.3
Calcium (mg)	6.9	22.6
Iron (mg)	2.2	2.7
Magnesium (mg)	15.2	29.5
Potassium (mg)	85.9	204
Zinc (mg)	0.6	0.95
Sodium (mg)	1.5	3.7

Portion 1 Cup

Number of Exchanges

Traditional Recipe
1 1/2 grain exchange
1/3 meat exchange (very lean)
1/3 starch exchange
3 fat exchange (2 PUFA, 1 MUFA)

Healthy Recipe
1 1/2 grain exchange
1 meat exchange (very lean)
1 starch exchange
1 2/3 fat exchange
(1/3 MUFA, 1 1/3 Omega-3-FA)
1/3 non-starchy vegetable exchange

Calories from Macronutrients

Protein   Carbohydrates   Fat

Traditional Recipe

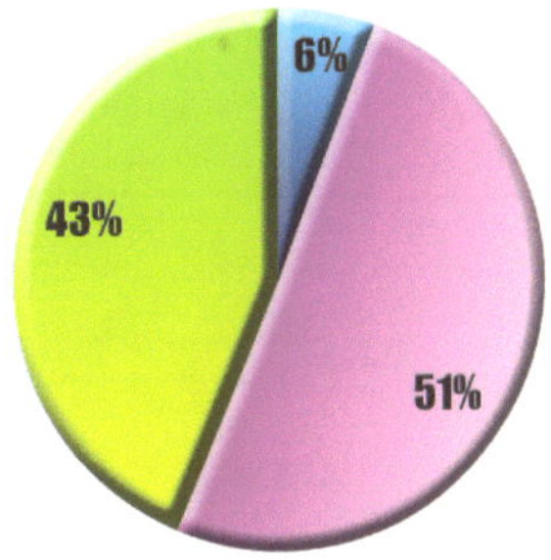

Healthy Recipe

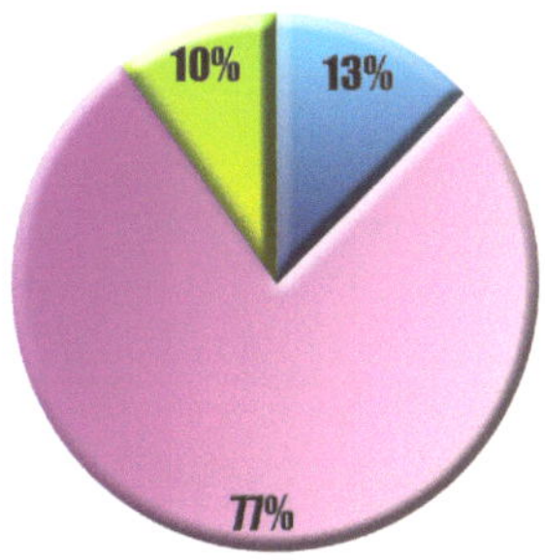

% Fiber Intake Compared to Average Daily Needs

Remaining Required Daily   Consumed

Traditional Recipe

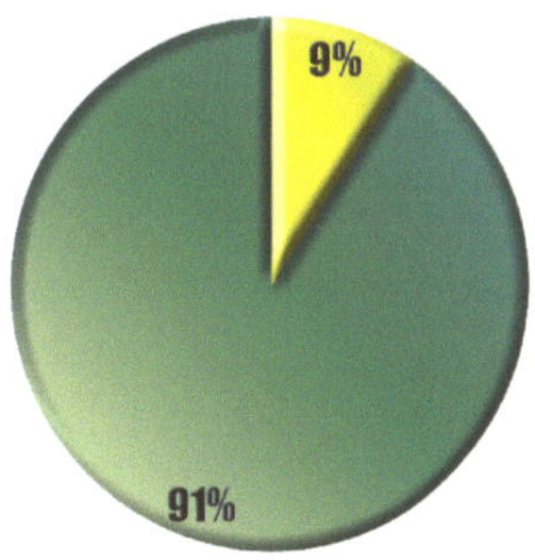

Healthy Recipe

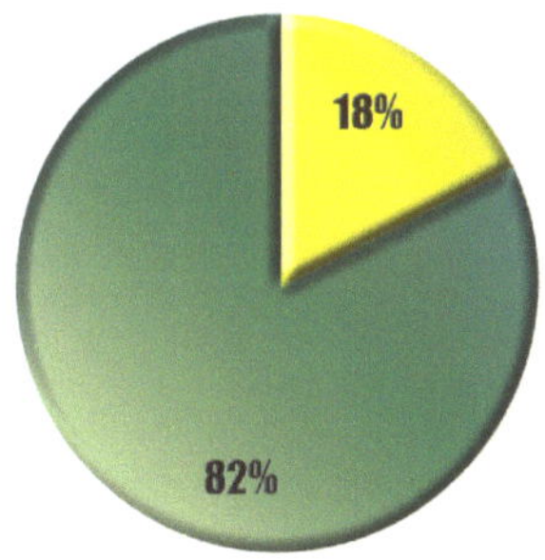

Recommended Portion Sizes & Meal Combinations

Traditional Recipe
(Calorie Controlled)

Men
1 1/2 cups of moa'adas
1 1/2 cups of traditional Dekous Eggplant

Women
1 cup of moa'adas
1 cup of traditional Dekous Eggplant

Healthy Recipe
(Calorie Controlled & Content Balanced)

Men
1 2/3 cups of moa'adas
2 cups of Dekous Eggplant
(see page:128)
1 cup of lowfat ayran

Women
1 cup of moa'adas
1 cup of Dekous Eggplant
(see page:128)
1 cup of lowfat ayran

Number of Exchanges in a Balanced Meal

Men
7 2/3 non-starchy vegetable exchange
6 3/4 fat exchange (4 1/2 MUFA, 2 1/4 Omega-3-FA)
2/3 meat exchange (very lean)
2/3 starch exchange
2 1/3 grain exchange
1 milk exchange

Women
4 non-starchy vegetable exchange
3 2/3 fat exchange
(2 1/3 MUFA, 1 1/3 Omega-3-FA)
1/3 meat exchange (very lean)
1/3 starch exchange
1 1/2 grain exchange
1 milk exchange

Rice Cooked with Eggplant

(Maklouba)

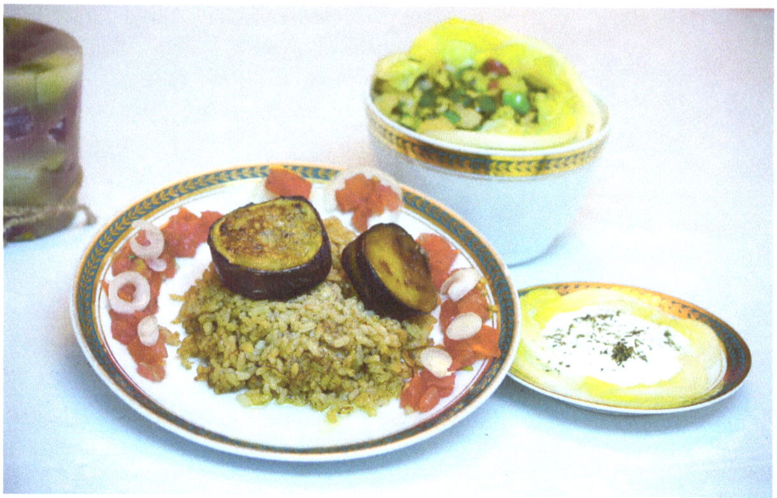

Traditional Recipe, 4 Servings, 4 Cups:

1 2/3 cups Thick Sliced Eggplant~154g
3/4 cup Red Tomato Slices~210g
1 cup Short White Rice Unenriched~219.92g
2 1/2 Tablespoons Corn Oil~34g
4 cups Water

Traditional Method of Preparation:

- Wash rice under running water, until water is clear; soak rice in cold water for 10 minutes
- Heat oil in a large frying pan, add sliced eggplant and fry over high heat for 5 minutes. Turn eggplant care fully with blunt ended tongs to brown evenly
- When lightly browned, transfer eggplant to cooking pan filled with 3 cups of water
- Fry tomato slices over high heat for 2 minutes
- Combine fried tomatoes with fried eggplant and water; bring it to a gentle boil for 8 minutes
- Transfer eggplant and tomatoes to a separate dish; cook rice in water instead of eggplant and tomatoes
- Cook over medium heat for 15 minutes
- On a serving plate, serve cooked rice and top it with fried tomatoes and eggplant
- Ready to serve

Healthy Recipe, 4 Servings, 4 Cups:

2 3/4 cups Thick Sliced Eggplant~260.68g
1 3/4 cups Red Tomato Slices~430.92g
2/3 cup Short Rice Unenriched~146.3g
4 teaspoons Corn Oil~18g
2 2/3 teaspoons Ground Flaxseed~6.65g
10 1/2 cups Water

Healthy Method of Preparation:

- Wash rice under running water, until water is clear; soak rice in warm water for 15 minutes
- In a cooking pan, bring 10 cups of water to gentle boil, add eggplant and tomatoes and cook over medium heat for 20 minutes
- Transfer eggplant and tomatoes to a separate dish; set aside
- Cook rice in water instead of eggplant and tomatoes; cook over medium heat for 15 minutes
- Reduce heat, cover and cook over low heat for another 4 minutes
- Turn stove off; sprinkle flaxseed and stir twice
- On serving plate, place serve cooked rice, top it with tomatoes and eggplant; brush eggplant with corn oil from upper layer
- Ready to serve

Nutritional Goal

The purpose of modification is to reduce calories and to enrich food with fiber. The calorie content of the healthy recipe is reduced by half, and fiber content is increased by more than 35%. Macronutrients of the healthy recipe are more balanced than macronutrients of the traditional recipe. The change in cooking method reduces the amount of oil absorbed by vegetables and preserves fat quality. This technique also keeps larger volume of foods leading to more pleasurable taste and earlier satiety feeling. The nutritional analysis shows that this modification adds more potassium, magnesium, calcium, vitamin A, and vitamin C to the healthy recipe when compared to the traditional recipe. The healthy recipe is recommended to individuals with malnutrition, excessive body weight, constipation, and high lipid profiles.

Nutrient Content	Traditional Recipe	Healthy Recipe
Portion	1 cup	1 cup
Weight (g)	193	232.75
Kilocalories (kcal)	556.2	214.8
Protein (g)	4.4	4.3
Carbohydrate (g)	47.7	37.33
Fat (g)	39	5.75
Saturated Fat (g)	5	0.76
Monounsaturated Fat (g)	9.5	1.34
Polyunsaturated Fat (g)	22.8	3.4
Trans Fatty Acid (g)	0.11	0.013
Cholesterol (g)	0	0
Omega-6 Linoleic (g)	22.4	2.8
Omega-3 Linolenic (g)	0.3	0.43
Fiber (g)	3.5	4.97
Sugar (g)	2.3	4.4
Water (L)	7.4	5.13
Thiamin (mg)	0.35	0.29
Riboflavin (mg)	0.1	0.06
Niacin (mg)	2.8	2.62
Vitamin B6 (mg)	0.1	0.15
Vitamin B12 (mcg)	0	0
Folate (DFE) mcg	143.3	116.4
Vitamin C (mg)	7.5	15
Vitamin D (mcg)	0	0
Vitamin A (RAE) (mcg)	135.7	277.6
Vitamin E (mg)	6.7	1.1
Calcium (mg)	10.36	21.9
Iron (mg)	2.6	2.1
Magnesium (mg)	23.8	35.87
Potassium (mg)	254.7	446
Zinc (mg)	0.76	0.76
Sodium (mg)	3.9	7.6

Portion 1 Cup

Number of Exchanges

Traditional Recipe
2/3 non-starchy vegetable exchange
2 grain exchange
2 fat exchange (PUFA)

Healthy Recipe
1 non-starchy vegetable exchange
1 1/4 grain exchange
1 2/3 fat exchange
(1 PUFA, 2/3 Omega-3-FA)

Calories from Macronutrients

Protein Carbohydrates Fat

Traditional Recipe

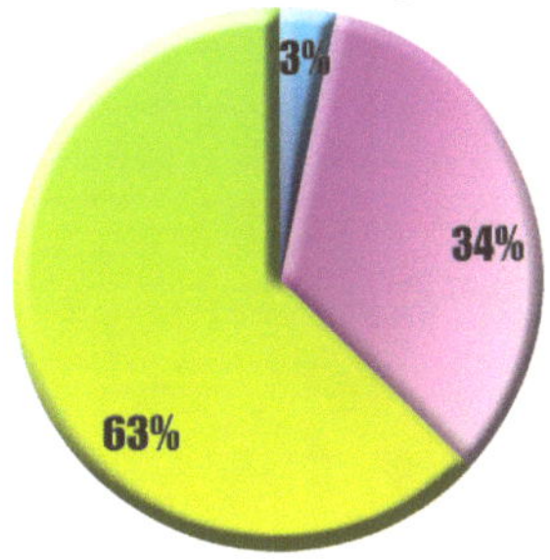

Healthy Recipe

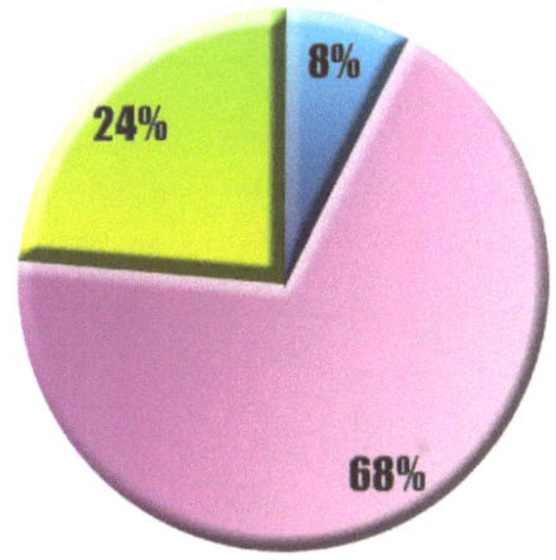

% Fiber Intake Compared to Average Daily Needs

Remaining Required Daily Consumed

Traditional Recipe

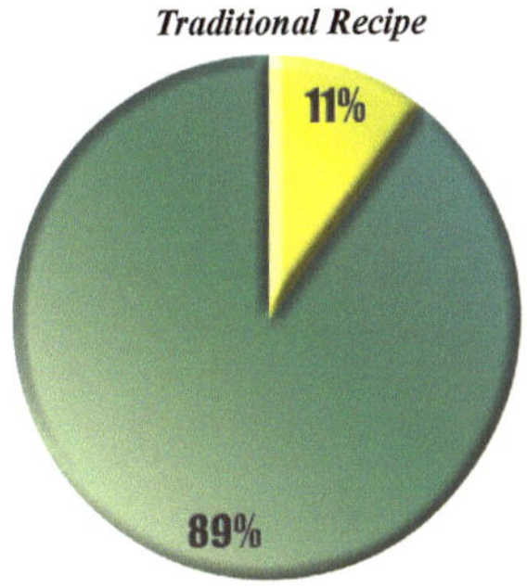

Healthy Recipe

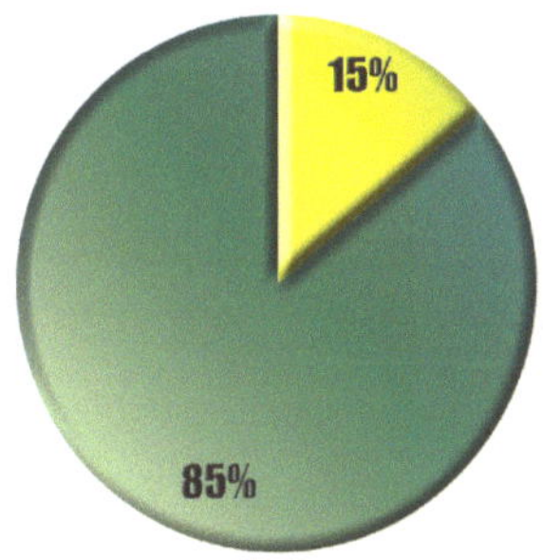

Recommended Portion Sizes & Meal Combinations

Traditional Recipe
(Calorie Controlled)

Men
1 1/4 cups of Maklouba
2/3 cup of regular plain yogurt

Women
2/3 cup of Maklouba
2/3 cup of regular plain yogurt

Healthy Recipe
(Calorie Controlled & Content Balanced)

Men
2 1/2 cups of Maklouba
1 1/2 cups of green salad-drizzled with olive oil
3/4 cup of lowfat plain yogurt

Women
1 1/3 cups of Maklouba
1 cup of green salad-drizzled with olive oil
2/3 cup of lowfat plain yogurt

Number of Exchanges in a Balanced Meal

Men
4 1/3 non-starchy vegetable exchange
3 grain exchange
5 1/2 fat exchange (2 1/2 PUFA, 1 1/2 MUFA, 1 1/2 Omega-3-FA)
1 1/4 milk exchange

Women
2 1/2 non-starchy vegetable exchange
1 2/3 grain exchange
3 fat exchange (1 1/3 PUFA, 1MUFA, 3/4 Omega-3-FA)
1 milk exchange

Rice Cooked with Fava Beans

(Arouz Be Al-foul)

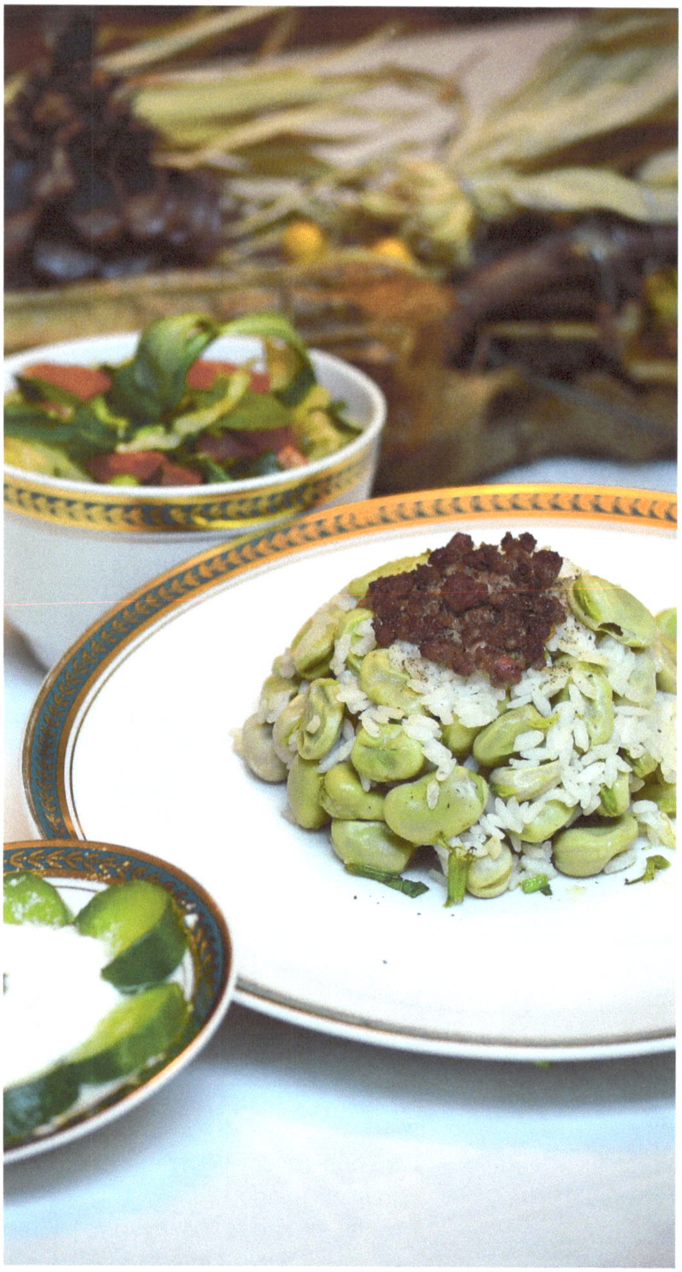

Traditional Recipe, 4 Servings, 4 Cups:

1 cup White Rice Unenriched~212.8g
2/3 cup Fresh Fava Beans~126.4g
3 1/4 Tablespoons Corn Oil~43.52g
4 cups Water

Traditional Method of Preparation:

- Wash rice under running water; soak in 1 cup of tap water for 10 minutes
- In a cooking pan, heat corn oil and fry beans over medium heat for 2 minutes
- Add rice to pan; stir for 1 minute
- Add 3 cups of water; cook over medium heat for 15 minutes
- Reduce heat, cover and cook over low heat for 5 minutes
- Ready to serve

Healthy Recipe, 4 Servings, 4 Cups:

3/4 cup Short White Rice Unenriched~172g
1 1/2 cup Fresh Fava Beans~302.5g
1/2 cup Chopped Onions~83.35g
3/4 cup Meat Broth~175.39g
4 3/4 cups Water

Healthy Method of Preparation:

- Wash rice until water is clear in the bowl; drain and soak rice in 2 cups of warm water for 10 minutes
- In a cooking pan, place chopped onions with 3/4 cup of water, and cook over medium heat for 5 minutes
- Add beans and meat broth. Stir over medium heat for 4 minutes
- Add rice and 2 cups of cold water, continue to cook over medium heat for 15 minutes
- Reduce heat, cover and continue to cook over low heat for 5 minutes
- Ready to serve

Nutritional Goal

The modification aims to substitute calories from fat for healthier calories, to improve fat quality, and to enrich food with fiber and nutrients. The change of proportion of rice to fava beans from 1.5:1 to 1:2 increases the nutritional values of food with a more enjoyable taste. Calories from fat are substituted with calories from protein leading to 17% increase in protein calories, 20% reduction in fat calories, and 10% savings of total calories. A comparison between nutritional analysis of the traditional and the healthy recipes shows that the healthy recipe has higher levels of different nutrients. Fiber content of the healthy recipe is increased by half, when compared to fiber content of the traditional recipe. Also, calcium content is increased by more than 200%, vitamin C is increased by more than 120%, and iron is increased by more than 20% in the healthy recipe as compared to the traditional recipe. The healthy recipe is recommended to individuals with constipation, osteoporosis, excessive body weight, and high lipid profiles.

Nutrient Content	Traditional Recipe	Healthy Recipe
Portion	1 cup	1 cup
Weight (g)	136	210
Kilocalories (kcal)	309.4	281.7
Protein (g)	5.228	16.3
Carbohydrate (g)	45.8	43.9
Fat (g)	11.35	4.06
Saturated Fat (g)	1.49	1.1
Monounsaturated Fat (g)	2.722	1.42
Polyunsaturated Fat (g)	6.56	1.05
Trans Fatty Acid (g)	0.03	0
Cholesterol (g)	0	26.4
Omega-6 Linoleic (g)	6.35	0.09
Omega-3 Linolenic (g)	0.146	0.19
Fiber (g)	2.7	4.5
Sugar (g)	0.57	2.2
Water (L)	7.09	34.9
Thiamin (mg)	0.36	0.38
Riboflavin (mg)	0.06	0.16
Niacin (mg)	2.662	5.54
Vitamin B6 (mg)	0.012	0.21
Vitamin B12 (mcg)	0	0.123
Folate (DFE) mcg	122.9	102.32
Vitamin C (mg)	10.43	26.39
Vitamin D (mcg)	0	0
Vitamin A (RAE) (mcg)	33.5	92.52
Vitamin E (mg)	1.84	0.16
Calcium (mg)	8.55	27.838
Iron (mg)	2.85	3.88
Magnesium (mg)	24.25	44.7
Potassium (mg)	119.4	303.44
Zinc (mg)	0.77	1.5
Sodium (mg)	16.33	252

Portion 1 Cup

Number of Exchanges

Traditional Recipe
2 grain exchange
2 1/3 fat exchange (PUFA)
1/3 starch
1/3 meat exchange (very lean)

Healthy Recipe
1 1/2 grain exchange
3/4 starch exchange
3/4 meat exchange (very lean)

Calories from Macronutrients

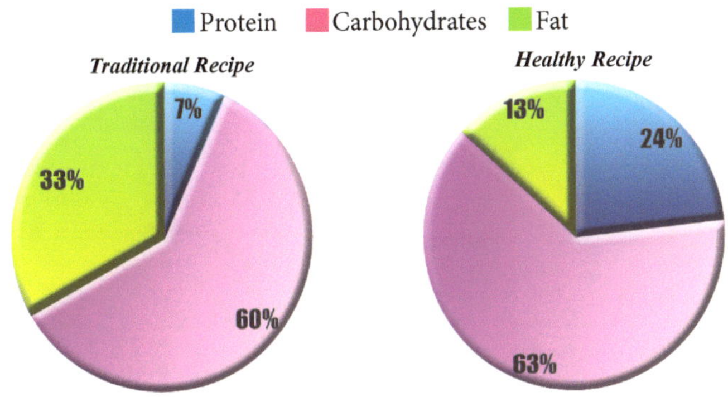

% Fiber Intake Compared to Average Daily Needs

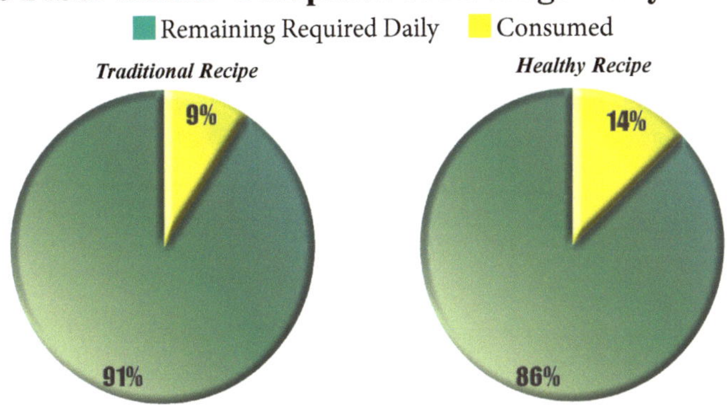

Recommended Portion Sizes & Meal Combinations

Traditional Recipe
(Calorie Controlled)

Men
1 1/2 cups of arouz be al-foul
1 1/2 cups of green salad
2/3 cup of meat and broth
1 cup of plain low fat yogurt

Women
1 cup of arouz be al-foul
1 cup of green salad
2/3 cup of plain low fat yogurt

Healthy Recipe
(Calorie Controlled & Content Balanced)

Men
1 2/3 cups of arouz be al-foul
1 1/2 cups of green salad-drizzled with olive oil
2/3 cup of meat & broth
1 cup of plain low fat yogurt

Women
1 cup of arouz be al-foul
1 cup of green salad-drizzled with olive oil
1/3 cup of meat & broth
2/3 cup of plain low fat yogurt

Number of Exchanges in a Balanced Meal

Men
1 1/4 starch
2 1/3 grain
2 1/4 meat exchange (1 1/4 very lean, 1 high fat)
1 3/4 non-starchy vegetable exchange
1 1/2 fat exchange (MUFA)
1 2/3 milk exchange

Women 33
3/4 starch exchange
1 1/2 grain exchange
3/4 meat exchange (very lean)
1 non-starchy vegetable exchange
1 fat exchange (MUFA)
1 milk exchange

Rice Cooked with Green Peas

(Arouz Be Al-Bazala'a)

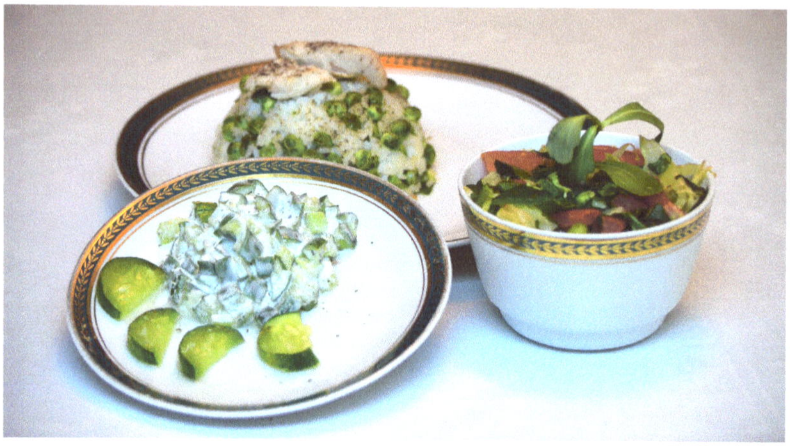

Traditional Recipe, 4 Servings, 4 Cups:

1 cup Unenriched Short Rice~240g
1 cup Green Peas~220g
1/3 cup Corn Oil~78g
2 3/4 cups Water

Traditional Method of Preparation:

- Wash and drain rice; soak rice in cold water for 10 minutes
- In a cooking pan, heat oil and fry peas over medium heat for 3 minutes
- Combine rice with peas and continue frying for 2 minutes Stir constantly to prevent sticking
- Add 2 3/4 cups of water, and cook over medium heat for 20 minutes
- Reduce heat, cover and cook over low heat for another 5 minutes
- Ready to serve

Healthy Recipe, 4 Servings, 4 Cups:

3/4 cup Unenriched Short Rice~187g
1 3/4 cups Green Peas~340g
1/4 cup Meat Broth~68g
7 Tablespoons Chopped Onions~68g
2 cups Water

Healthy Method of Preparation:

- Wash rice under running water; soak in warm water for 20 minutes
- In a cooking pan, combine onions with 1/4 cup of water and bring to boil over medium heat for 3 minutes
- Add rice, peas, 2 cups of water, and meat broth with onions, and cook over medium heat for 15 minutes
- Cover and cook over low heat for 5 minutes
- Ready to serve

Nutritional Goal

The modification aims to reduce calories and to enrich food with fiber and micronutrients. The calorie content of the healthy recipe is reduced by more than 30% when compared to the calorie content of the traditional recipe. Despite the calories from carbohydrate are predominant in the healthy recipe, most of the carbohydrate comes from peas that make the healthy recipe a good choice to individuals with high lipid profiles. The change in the ratio of rice: peas and the addition of onions enrich the food with fiber. The healthy recipe contains 25% more fiber when compared to fiber content of the traditional recipe. Thus, it helps individuals with high lipid profile, constipation, and bloating problems. This food is served with meat or chicken, because these foods contain hidden fat, thus amount of fat used in preparation is reduced. The nutritional analysis shows that the healthy recipe contains more calcium, magnesium, potassium, zinc, B complex, vitamin A, and vitamin C, when compared to their levels in the traditional recipe.

Nutrient Content	Traditional Recipe	Healthy Recipe
Portion	1 cup	1 cup
Weight (g)	224	222
Kilocalories (kcal)	441	275.1
Protein (g)	6.9	11.5
Carbohydrate (g)	56.8	52
Fat (g)	20	1.8
Saturated Fat (g)	2.6	0.5
Monounsaturated Fat (g)	4.9	0.6
Polyunsaturated Fat (g)	11.8	0.5
Trans Fatty Acid (g)	0.05	0
Cholesterol (g)	0	10.6
Omega-6 Linoleic (g)	11.58	0.07
Omega-3 Linolenic (g)	0.16	0.046
Fiber (g)	4.8	6.24
Sugar (g)	3.3	5.7
Water (L)	8.14	18
Thiamin (mg)	0.48	0.5
Riboflavin (mg)	0.11	0.17
Niacin (mg)	3.6	4.7
Vitamin B6 (mg)	0.12	0.27
Vitamin B12 (mcg)	0	0.05
Folate (DFE) mcg	175.7	166
Vitamin C (mg)	7.87	13.6
Vitamin D (mcg)	0	0
Vitamin A (RAE) (mcg)	134.52	213.1
Vitamin E (mg)	3.5	0.35
Calcium (mg)	16.79	30.6
Iron (mg)	3.43	3.6
Magnesium (mg)	35.6	47.8
Potassium (mg)	196.48	314.9
Zinc (mg)	1.33	1.8
Sodium (mg)	2.27	89.4

Portion 1 Cup

Number of Exchanges

Traditional Recipe
2 grain exchange
1/2 starch exchange
1/2 meat exchange (very lean)
4 1/3 fat exchange (PUFA)

Healthy Recipe
1 1/2 grain exchange
1 starch exchange
1 meat exchange (very lean)

Calories from Macronutrients

Protein · Carbohydrates · Fat

Traditional Recipe

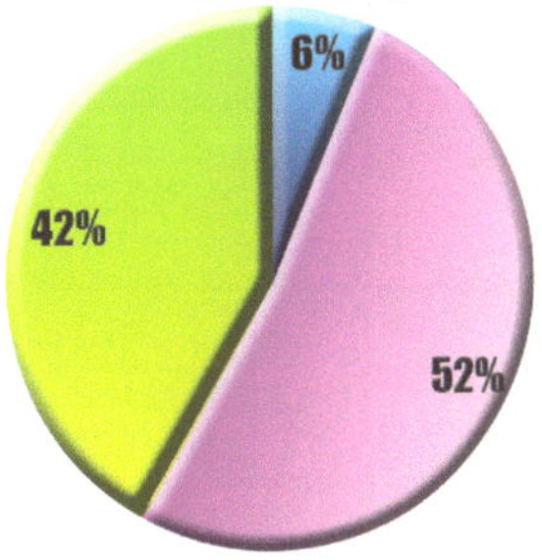

Healthy Recipe

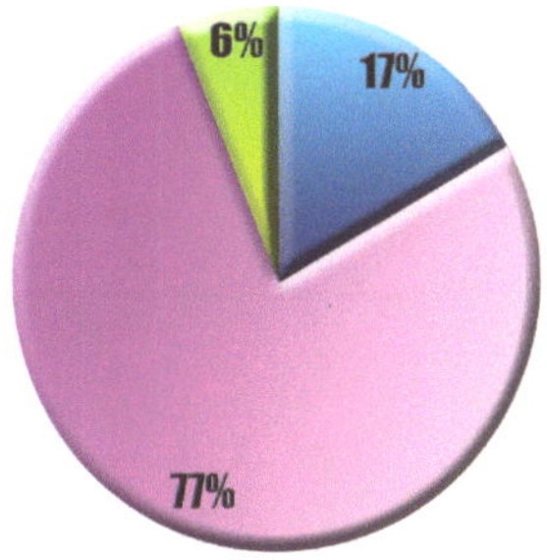

% Fiber Intake Compared to Average Daily Needs

Remaining Required Daily · Consumed

Traditional Recipe

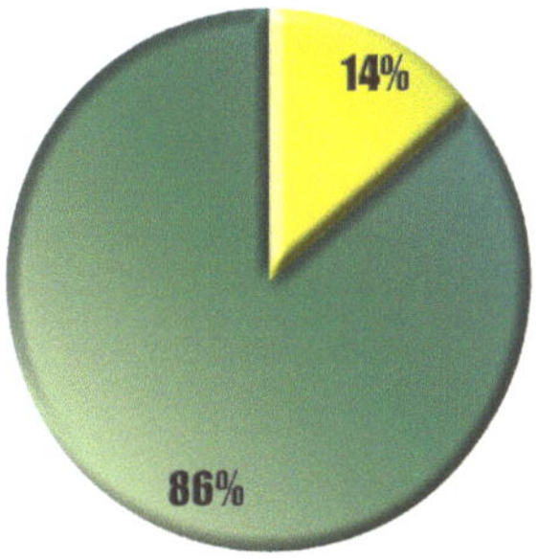

Healthy Recipe

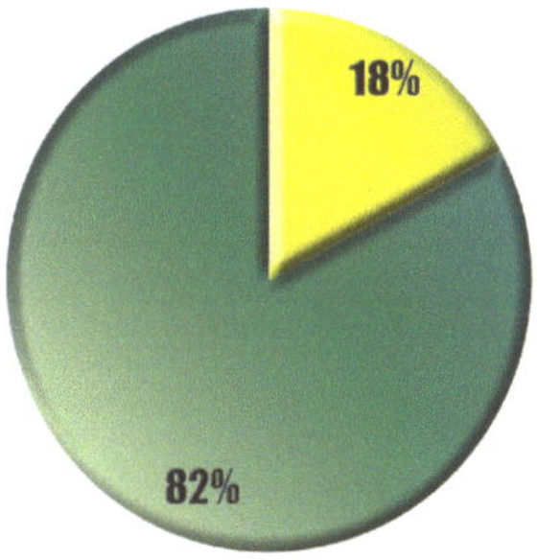

Recommended Portion Sizes & Meal Combinations

Traditional Recipe
(Calorie Controlled)

Men
1 1/4 cups of arouz be al bazazala'a
1 1/4 cups of cucumber yogurt salad
1 cup of shank and broth

Women
3/4 cup of arouz be al-bazala'a
1 cup of cucumber yogurt salad
2/3 cup of shank and broth

Healthy Recipe
(Calorie Controlled & Content Balanced)

Men
1 3/4 cups of arouz be al-bazala'a
1 cup of cucumber yogurt salad
(see page:!28)
2/3 cup of lean shank and broth
2 1/2 cups of green salad-drizzled with vinegar

Women
1 cup of arouz be al-bazala'a
1 cup of cucumber yogurt salad
(see page:128)
1/3 cup of lean shank and broth
2 cups of green salad-drizzled with vinegar

Number of Exchanges in a Balanced Meal

Men
2 2/3 grain exchange
1 1/3 starch exchange
1 milk exchange
3 1/3 non-starchy vegetable exchange
3 1/3 meat exchange
(2 medium fat, 1 1/3 very lean)

Women
1 1/2 grain exchange
1 starch exchange
1 milk exchange
2 3/4 non-starchy vegetable exchange
2 meat exchange
(1 medium fat, 1 very lean meat)

Rice Cooked with Mushrooms

(Arouz Be Al-Fotour)

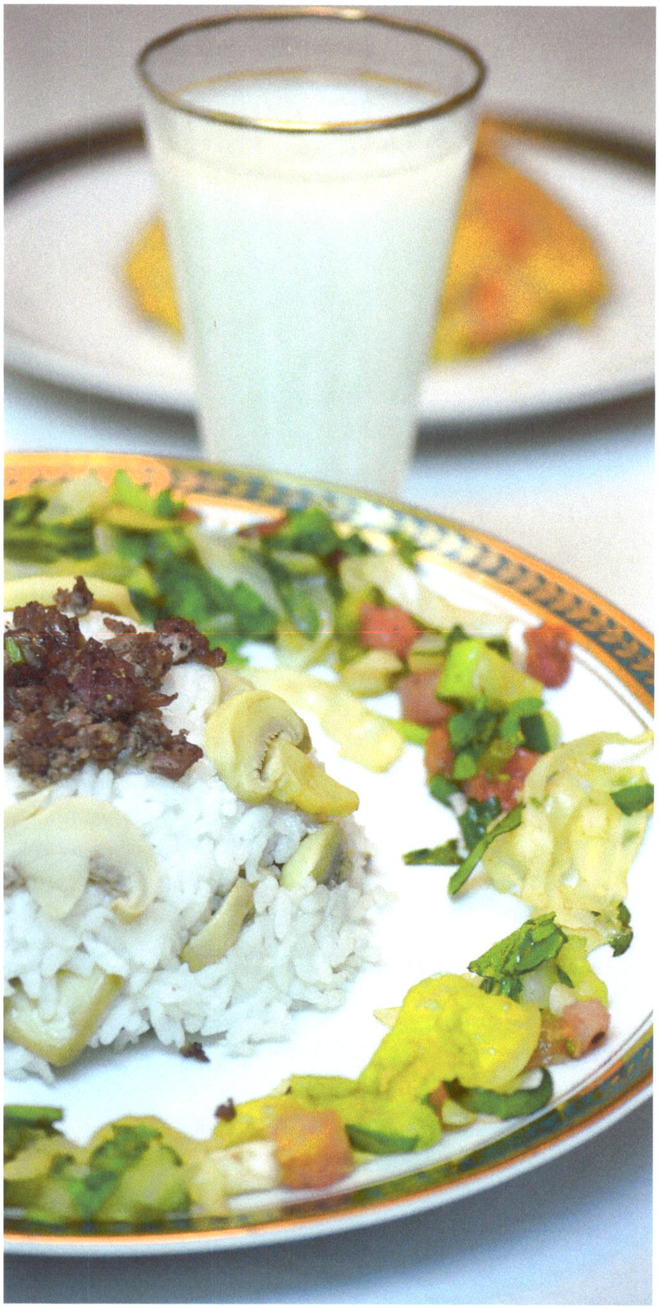

Traditional Recipe, 4 Servings, 4 Cups:

3/4 cup Short Rice Unenriched~179g
1 1/3 cups Sliced Mushrooms~313.6g
2 1/3 Tablespoons Corn Oil~32g
2 cups Water

Traditional Method of Preparation:

- Wash rice under running water; soak in water for 10 minutes
- In a cooking pan, heat oil and fry mushroom over medium heat for 2 minutes
- Combine rice with mushrooms; stir for 2 minutes
- Add 2 cups of water; cook over medium heat for another 20 minutes
- Reduce heat, cover, and simmer over low heat for additional 5 minutes
- Ready to serve

Healthy Recipe, 4 Servings, 4 Cups:

3/4 cup Short Rice Unenriched~167g
1 1/2 cups Sliced Mushrooms~340g
1 1/2 teaspoons Corn Oil~6.98g
1 1/2 teaspoons Flaxseed~3.79g
1/3 cup Chopped Onions~60.72g
1 3/4 cups Water

Healthy Method of Preparation:

- Wash rice until water is clear; drain
- Soak rice with 2 cups of warm water for 15 minutes
- In a cooking pan, combine chopped onions with 1/3 cup of water and bring to boil over medium heat for 5 minutes, until onions are juicy and thick
- Combine mushroom, rice, 1 1/2 cups of water, and onions; stir twice, and continue to cook over medium heat for 15 minutes
- Reduce heat and add corn oil and flaxseed; cover and cook over low heat for another 5 minutes
- Ready to serve

Nutritional Goal

The modification aims to reduce calorie content, to improve quality of fat, and to enrich food with fiber. The calorie content of the healthy recipe is reduced by more than 25% when compared to the calorie content of the traditional recipe. The quality of fat content in the healthy recipe is also improved since total fat and saturated fat are reduced by more than 70%, when Omega-3-FA is increased by more than 190%, when compared to the traditional recipe. The nutritional analysis shows that the healthy recipe is enriched with fiber, calcium, magnesium, potassium, and zinc when compared to nutrient contents of the traditional recipe. The healthy recipe is recommended to individuals with heart disease, high lipid profiles, excessive body weight, and post-menopausal women.

Nutrient Content	Traditional Recipe	Healthy Recipe
Portion	1 cup	1 cup
Weight (g)	220.4	201.89
Kilocalories (kcal)	276.19	197.3
Protein (g)	4.4	4.6
Carbohydrate (g)	39.4	39.1
Fat (g)	11.34	2.6
Saturated Fat (g)	1.5	0.35
Monounsaturated Fat (g)	2.7	0.56
Polyunsaturated Fat (g)	6.5	1.44
Trans Fatty Acid (g)	0.03	0.005
Cholesterol (g)	0	0
Omega-6 Linoleic (g)	6.4	1.09
Omega-3 Linolenic (g)	0.08	0.24
Fiber (g)	3	3.67
Sugar (g)	1.7	2.6
Water (L)	6	5.7
Thiamin (mg)	0.32	0.33
Riboflavin (mg)	0.04	0.04
Niacin (mg)	3.1	3.11
Vitamin B6 (mg)	0.13	0.1
Vitamin B12 (mcg)	0	0
Folate (DFE) mcg	113	110.3
Vitamin C (mg)	0	0.97
Vitamin D (mcg)	0	0
Vitamin A (RAE) (mcg)	0	0.1
Vitamin E (mg)	1.9	0.41
Calcium (mg)	10	16.34
Iron (mg)	2.5	2.5
Magnesium (mg)	15.35	27.6
Potassium (mg)	113	170.7
Zinc (mg)	0.7	1.1
Sodium (mg)	334	361.9

Portion 1 Cup

Number of Exchanges

Traditional Recipe
1 1/2 grain exchange
1/3 non-starchy vegetable exchange
1 3/4 fat exchange (PUFA)

Healthy Recipe
1 1/2 grain exchange
1/2 non-starchy vegetable exchange
2/3 fat exchange
(1/3 PUFA, 1/3 Omega-3-FA)

Calories from Macronutrients

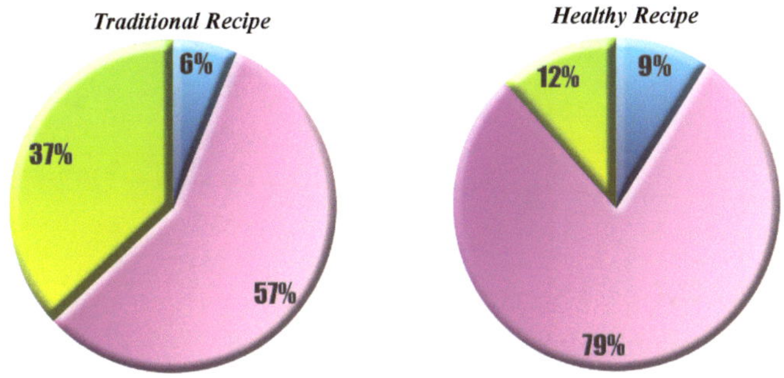

% Fiber Intake Compared to Average Daily Needs

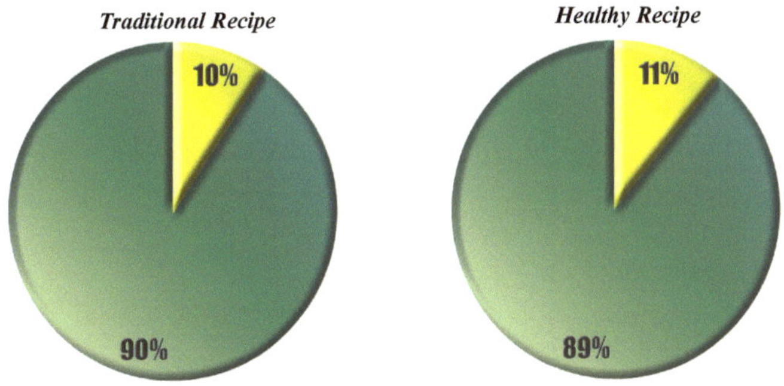

Recommended Portion Sizes & Meal Combinations

Traditional Recipe
(Calorie Controlled)

Men
2 1/4 cups of arouz be al-fotour
2/3 cup of regular plain yogurt
1 cup of shank and broth

Women
1 1/3 cups of arouz be al-fotour
2/3 cup of regular plain yogurt
2/3 cup of shank and broth

Healthy Recipe
(Calorie Controlled & Content Balanced)

Men
2 3/4 cups of arouz be al-fotour
2/3 cup of shank and broth
2 1/2 cups of green salad-drizzled with vinegar
2/3 cup of lowfat plain yogurt

Women
1 2/3 cups of arouz be al-fotour
1/3 cup of shank and broth
1 1/2 cups of green salad-drizzled with vinegar
2/3 cup of lowfat plain yogurt

Number of Exchanges in a Balanced Meal

Men
4 grain exchange
3 3/4 non-starchy vegetable exchange
2 fat exchange (1 PUFA, 1 Omega-3-FA)
1 milk exchange
2 meat exchange (high fat)

Women
2 1/3 grain exchange
2 1/4 non-starchy vegetable exchange
1 fat exchange
(2/3 PUFA, 1/2 Omega-3-FA)
1 milk exchange
1 meat exchange (high fat)

Spiced Rice
(Makbous-Kabsah)

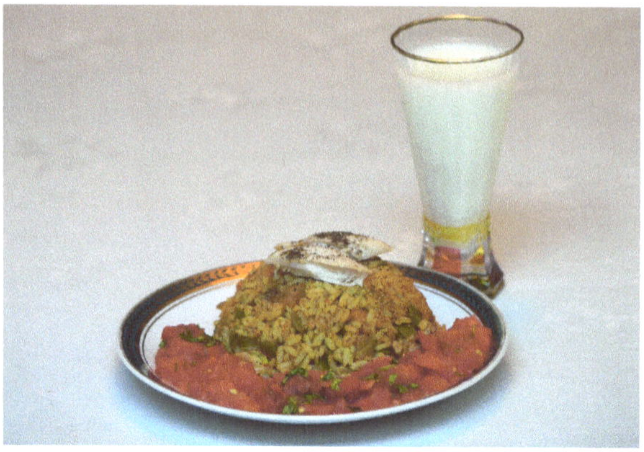

Traditional Recipe, 4 Servings, 4 Cups:

1 cup Medium Rice Unenriched~180g
1/2 cup Chopped Green Peppers~69g
1/3 cup Chopped Red Tomatoes~324g
1/4 cup Chopped Onions~35.4g
2/3 Tablespoon Ground Cardamom~4.3g
1/2 Tablespoon Ground Garlic~6.9g
2/3 Tablespoon Tomato Paste~9.3g
3 1/2 Tablespoons Corn Oil~46.6g
1 1/2 cups Water

Traditional Method of Preparation:

- Wash and drain rice; soak rice in cold water for 10 minutes
- Heat oil and fry onions over medium heat for 3 minutes
- Combine green peppers, red tomatoes and garlic
- Continue frying for another 5 minutes; stir constantly to prevent sticking
- Place the remaining ingredients together with 1 1/2 cups of water and cook over medium heat for another 20 minutes
- Reduce heat, cover and cook over low heat for another 5 minutes
- Ready to serve

Healthy Recipe, 4 Servings, 4 Cups:

1/2 cup Medium Rice Unenriched~93.7g
1 3/4 cups Chopped Green Peppers~226g
1 3/4 cups Chopped Red Tomatoes~414g
1/2 cup Chopped Onions~72g
2/3 Tablespoon Ground Cardamom~4.5g
2/3 Tablespoon Ground Garlic~7.2g
3 1/4 Tablespoons Tomato Paste~52.28g
2/3 Tablespoon Ground Flaxseed~4.5g
4 cups Water

Healthy Method of Preparation:

- Wash rice under running water, until water is clear; soak rice in warm water for 20 minutes
- Bring 4 cups of water to boil, and combine green peppers, red tomatoes, onions, and garlic
- Cook over medium heat for 10 minutes
- Mix tomato paste, cardamom, flaxseed and continue cooking for another 3 minutes
- Add rice with cooked vegetables and cook over medium heat for 15 minutes
- Reduce heat, cover and cook over low heat for another 5 minutes
- Ready to serve

Nutritional Goal

The modification of this recipe is essential since it is widely consumed in the Middle East and Gulf regions. This modification aims to save calories, to condense food with nutrients, to improve quality of fat, and to boost the joyful taste of this meal. Calories of the healthy recipe are reduced by half the calories of the traditional recipe. Total fat and saturated fat are reduced by more than 80% when compared to their levels of the traditional recipe. The healthy recipe is also cholesterol and trans fatty acid free. Although the healthy recipe contains great amounts of carbohydrate, the proportion of complex carbohydrate to simple carbohydrate is 14:1. To change the ratio of non-starchy vegetables to rice, this enriches food with different nutrients, most importantly, fiber. The healthy recipe is enriched with more than 15% fiber. A comparison between the nutritional analysis of recipes shows that the healthy recipe contains higher levels of vitamin C, vitamin A, calcium, magnesium, and potassium. The sodium content of the healthy recipe is reduced by more than half as well. The omega-6: omega-3 ratio is improved from 69:1 in the traditional recipe, compared to 1:1 in the healthy recipe. The healthy recipe is recommended to individuals with heart disease, high lipid profiles, high blood pressure, constipation, bloating, osteoporosis, and obesity.

Nutrient Content	Traditional Recipe	Healthy Recipe
Portion	1 cup	1 cup
Weight (g)	228	205.2
Kilocalories (kcal)	293.4	133.5
Protein (g)	4.2	3.5
Carbohydrate (g)	42	28.7
Fat (g)	12.2	1
Saturated Fat (g)	1.6	0.17
Monounsaturated Fat (g)	2.9	0.2
Polyunsaturated Fat (g)	7	0.6
Trans Fatty Acid (g)	0.033	0
Cholesterol (g)	0	0
Omega-6 Linoleic (g)	6.9	0.17
Omega-3 Linolenic (g)	0.1	0.27
Fiber (g)	3.1	3.8
Sugar (g)	3.2	4.9
Water (L)	6.07	3.4
Thiamin (mg)	0.31	0.24
Riboflavin (mg)	0.1	0.1
Niacin (mg)	2.5	1.9
Vitamin B6 (mg)	0.14	0.3
Vitamin B12 (mcg)	0	0
Folate (DFE) mcg	119.8	80.3
Vitamin C (mg)	25.7	60.1
Vitamin D (mcg)	0	0
Vitamin A (RAE) (mcg)	234.5	324.4
Vitamin E (mg)	2.4	0.7
Calcium (mg)	21.2	31.1
Iron (mg)	2.4	1.7
Magnesium (mg)	25.7	32
Potassium (mg)	311.4	416
Zinc (mg)	0.8	0.7
Sodium (mg)	24	8.5

Portion 1 Cup

Number of Exchanges

Traditional Recipe
2 grain exchange
1/4 non-starchy vegetable exchange
2 1/2 fat exchange (PUFA)

Healthy Recipe
1 grain exchange
1 non-starchy vegetable exchange
1/2 fat exchange (Omega-3-FA)

Calories from Macronutrients

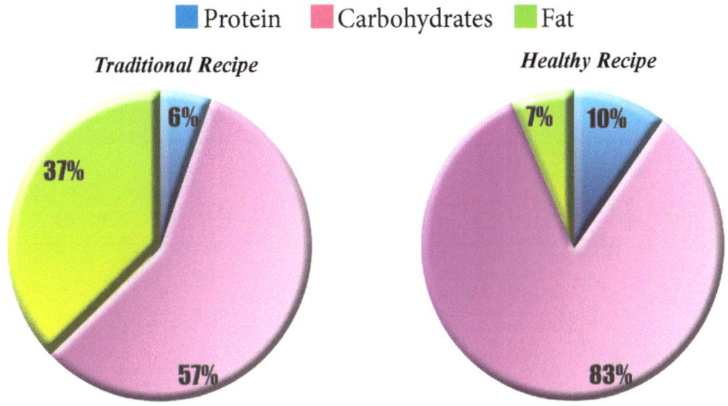

% Fiber Intake Compared to Average Daily Needs

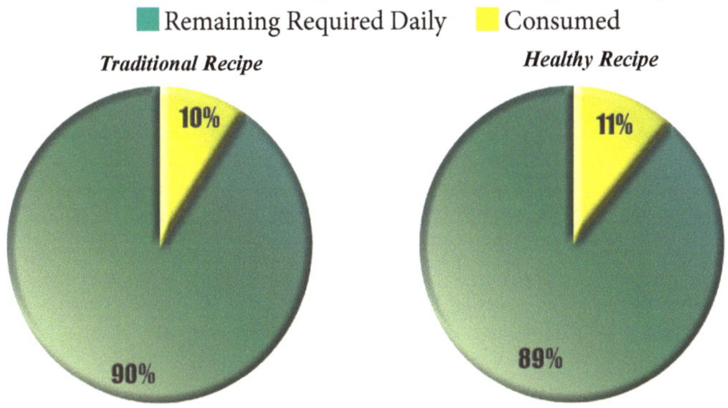

Recommended Portion Sizes & Meal Combinations

Traditional Recipe
(Calorie Controlled)

Men
1 1/2 cup of makbous-kabsah
1 serving of shank meat(3oz)
1 1/2 cup of tomato dekous
3/4 cup of regular plain yogurt

Women
3/4 cup of makbous-kabsah
2/3 serving of shank meat(2oz)
1 cup of tomato dekous
1/2 cup of regular plain yogurt

Healthy Recipe
(Calorie Controlled & Content Balanced)

Men
3 cup of makbous-kabsah
1 serving of lean shank meat(3oz)
2 cup of tomato dekous
3/4 cup of lowfat plain yogurt

Women
1 1/2 cup of makbous-kabsah
1 serving of lean shank meat(3oz)
1 cup of tomato dekous
1/2 cup of lowfat plain yogurt

Number of Exchanges in a Balanced Meal

Men
3 grain exchange
5 non-starchy vegetable exchange
1 1/2 fat exchange (Omega-3-FA)
3 meat exchange (lean)
1 1/4 milk exchange

Women
1 1/2 grain exchange
2 1/2 non-starchy vegetable exchange
3/4 fat exchange (Omega-3-FA)
3 meat exchange (lean)
1 milk exchange

Spiced Rice Cooked with Fish
(Sayadeyah)

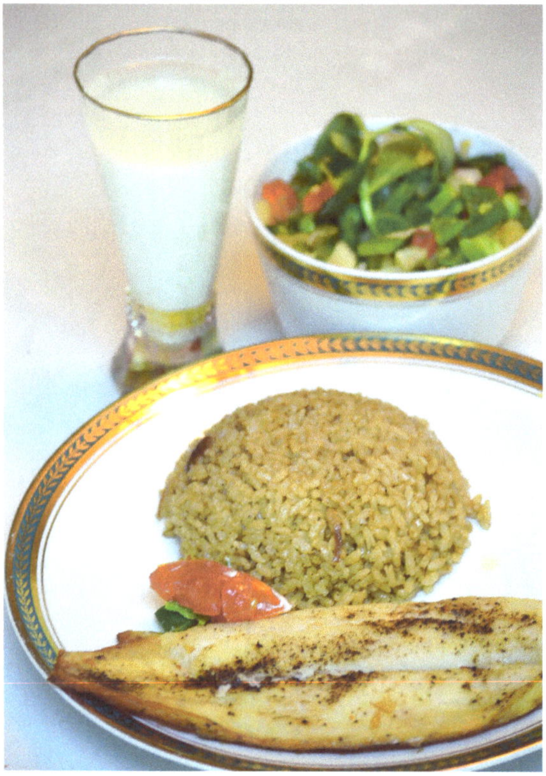

Traditional Recipe, 4 Servings, 4 Cups:

1 3/4 cups Shredded Onions~288g
1 1/2 teaspoons Ground Cardamom~3.75g
1 1/2 teaspoons Cumin~3g
1 1/2 teaspoons Black Pepper~3g
8 3/4 Tablespoons Corn Oil to Fry Onions~120.6g
3/4 cup Medium White Rice~162g
6 oz. Fish Fillet~171g
2 1/3 Tablespoons White Flour~18g
2 cups Water

Traditional Method of Preparation:

- Wash rice under running water, until water is clear
- Soak rice in water for 10 minutes
- In a cooking pan, heat 6 tablespoons of corn oil and fry onions over high heat for 10 minutes, until onions are dark brown.
- Add spices to fried onions; stir for 1 minute
- Combine rice and 2 cups of water with fried onions; continue to cook over medium heat for 20 minutes
- Turn stove off, and simmer for 5 minutes
- Coat fish with flour, and fry fish over high heat, until golden brown
- Ready to serve

Healthy Recipe, 4 Servings, 4 Cups:

1 1/4 cups Shredded Onions~205g
4 teaspoons Ground Cardamom~10g
1 teaspoon Cumin~2g
1 teaspoon Black Pepper~2g
2 1/2 teaspoons Corn Oil~11 g
2/3 cup Medium White Rice~130 g
9.5 oz. Fish Fillet~269g
1/2 cup Water

Healthy Method of Preparation:

- Wash rice under running water, until water is clear
- Soak rice in warm water for 20 minutes
- Brush pre-heated nonstick skillet with corn oil, brown onions over high heat for 20 minutes; stir frequently
- Add cumin, cardamom, and black pepper to onions; stir for 1 minute
- In a cooking pan, combine onions, rice with 1 1/2 cups of water and cook over medium heat for 15 minutes
- Turn stove off, and simmer for 5 minutes
- Pre-heat oven at high heat for 10 minutes
- Brush a baking pan with corn oil, place fish and bake in medium heat for 12 minutes
- Brush hot baked fish with corn oil
- Ready to serve

Nutritional Goal

The modification of this recipe is essential since fat is the predominant macronutrient in the traditional recipe, 60%. The modification aims to reduce calories, to balance calories from macronutrients, and to balance omega-6:omega-3 ratio. The calories provided by the healthy recipe are reduced by half when compared to calories provided by the traditional recipe. The healthy cooking method preserves the quality of fat; thus, the ratio of omega-6: omega-3 is healthier, 10:1, when compared to 53:1 of the traditional recipe. The trans fatty acid is nearly eliminated in the healthy recipe; it is reduced by more than 85%. Comparing to the traditional recipe, the reduction of fat, protein, and carbohydrate by more than 60%, 30%, and 50% respectively is a reason for more balanced calories from macronutrients in the healthy recipe. The nutritional analysis shows that healthy recipe is enriched with potassium and vitamin A, when there is no change in levels of most of other nutrients. Despite that fiber is reduced in the healthy recipe, the main source of fiber in the traditional recipe is white rice, which is a simple carbohydrate. The healthy recipe is highly suggested since it encourages the consumption of fish instead of red meat and is also recommended to individuals with excessive body weight.

Nutrient Content	Traditional Recipe	Healthy Recipe
Portion	1 cup	1 cup
Weight (g)	132	219.6
Kilocalories (kcal)	473	188.5
Protein (g)	11.2	7
Carbohydrate (g)	35	15
Fat (g)	32	7.2
Saturated Fat (g)	4.4	1.4
Monounsaturated Fat (g)	8.3	2.5
Polyunsaturated Fat (g)	18	3.06
Trans Fatty Acid (g)	0.1	0.008
Cholesterol (g)	23.5	37.3
Omega-6 Linoleic (g)	17	2
Omega-3 Linolenic (g)	0.32	0.19
Fiber (g)	1.4	0.8
Sugar (g)	3.3	2.2
Water (L)	0.3	0.3
Thiamin (mg)	0.3	0.2
Riboflavin (mg)	0.1	0.11
Niacin (mg)	1.8	0.6
Vitamin B6 (mg)	0.15	0.1
Vitamin B12 (mcg)	0	0
Folate (DFE) mcg	111	43.6
Vitamin C (mg)	4.6	3.3
Vitamin D (mcg)	0	0
Vitamin A (RAE) (mcg)	77.7	123.6
Vitamin E (mg)	5.2	0.8
Calcium (mg)	36	16.4
Iron (mg)	1.8	1
Magnesium (mg)	34.4	34
Potassium (mg)	280.3	318
Zinc (mg)	0.9	1
Sodium (mg)	82	38

Portion 1 Cup: 2 oz Fish, 1/3 Cup of Rice

Number of Exchanges

Traditional Recipe
6 3/4 fat exchange (PUFA)
1 1/2 grain exchange
1 1/3 meat exchange (lean)
1/3 non-starchy vegetable exchange

Healthy Recipe
2/3 fat exchange (PUFA)
1 1/4 grain exchange
2 meat exchange (lean)
1/3 non-starchy vegetable exchange

Calories from Macronutrients

Protein Carbohydrates Fat

Traditional Recipe

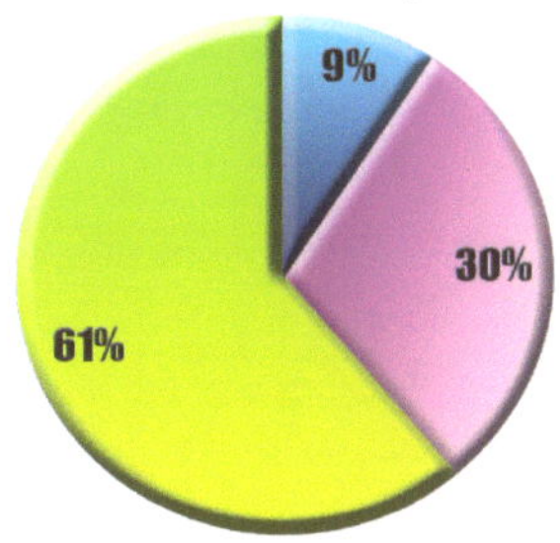

Healthy Recipe

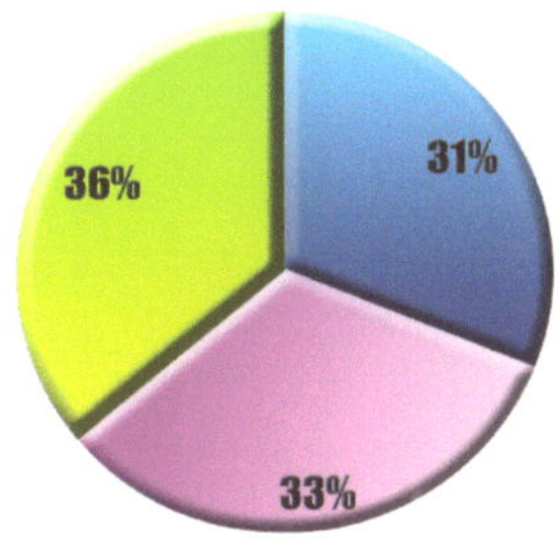

% Fiber Intake Compared to Average Daily Needs

Remaining Required Daily Consumed

Traditional Recipe

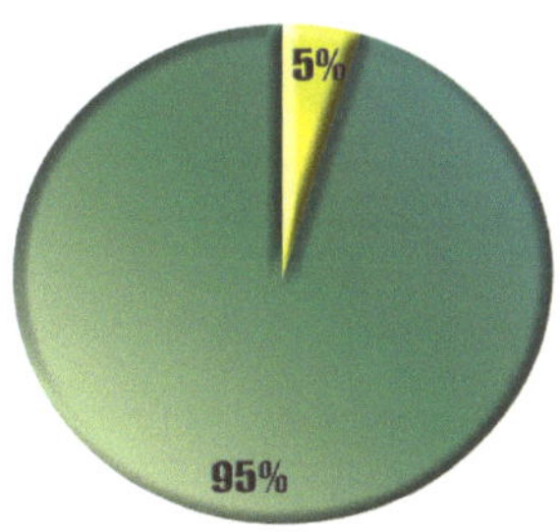

Healthy Recipe

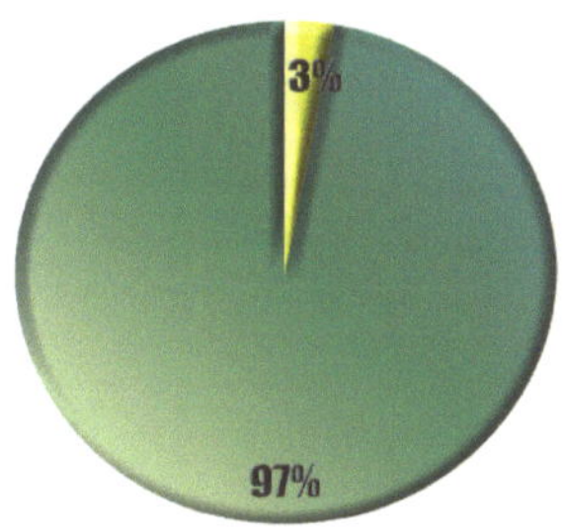

Recommended Portion Sizes & Meal Combinations

Traditional Recipe
(Calorie Controlled)

Men
1 1/4 cups of sayadeyah
2/3 serving of deep fried fish fillet

Women
3/4 cup of sayadeyah
1/3 serving of deep fried fish fillet

Healthy Recipe
(Calorie Controlled & Content Balanced)

Men
2 3/4 cups of sayadeyah
2 cups of green salad-drizzled with olive oil
1 cup of lowfat ayran

Women
1 cup of sayadeyah
1 1/2 serving of oven grilled fish fillet
1 1/2 cups of green salad-drizzled with olive oil
1 cup of lowfat ayran

Number of Exchanges in a Balanced Meal

Men
3 non-starchy vegetable exchange
3 2/3 fat exchange
(2 MUFA, 1 2/3 PUFA)
3 1/3 grain exchange
5 1/2 meat exchange (lean)
1 milk exchange

Women
2 non-starchy vegetable exchange
2 fat exchange (1 1/2 MUFA, 2/3 PUFA)
1 1/4 grain exchange
2 meat exchange (lean)
1 milk exchange

MEAT

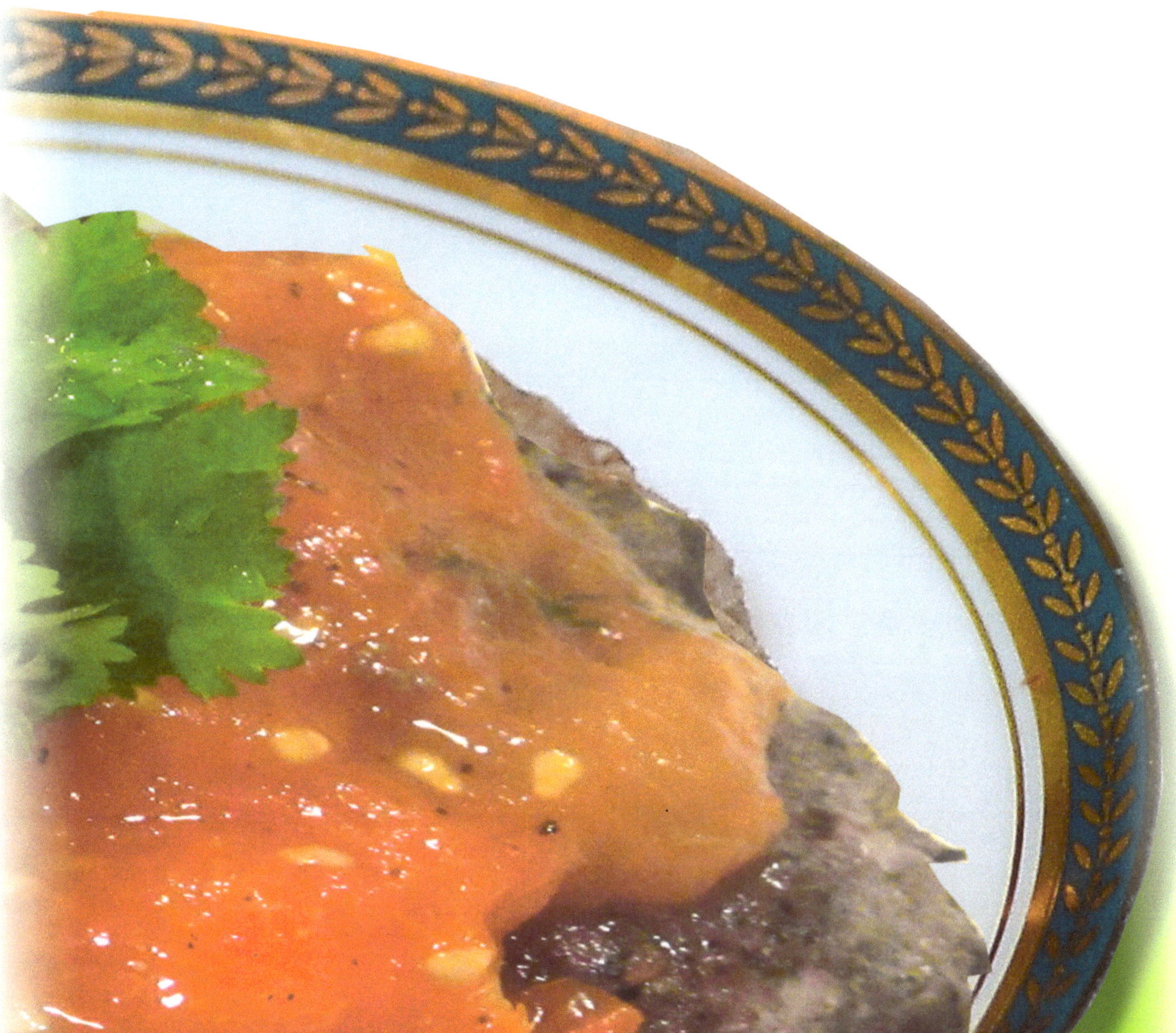

Meat Balls in Tomato Base

(Dawoud Basha)

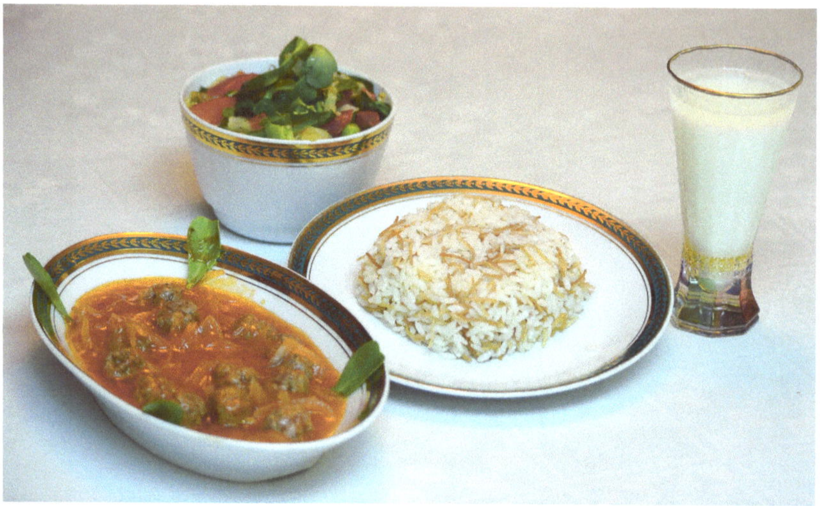

Traditional Recipe, 4 Servings, 4 Cups:

7.2 oz. Medium Fat Ground Meat~204g
3/4 cup Sliced Onion~141.6g
7 1/2 tablespoons Tomato Paste~118.08g
1 teaspoon Black Pepper~2g
3 3/4 Tablespoons Corn Oil~50.4g
4 cups Water

Traditional Method of Preparation:

- Season meat with black pepper
- Add 1/2 cup of water to meat; mix together until meat is moist and easy to shape
- Shape meat into balls
- Heat corn oil and fry onions over medium heat for 5 minutes, until onions are gold
- Combine meat balls with onions; cook for 10 minutes, until meat is brown; stir frequently
- Add 3 1/2 cups of water and tomato paste to pan; stir until water is red
- Cover and cook over moderate heat for another 10 minutes
- Ready to serve

Healthy Recipe, 4 Servings, 4 Cups:

3.2 oz. Lean Meat~93g
1 1/4 cups Sliced Onions~186.32g
3 Tablespoons Tomato Paste~50.58g
2 1/4 teaspoons Black Pepper~4.5g
2 1/3 teaspoons Ground Flaxseed~5.8g
1 1/2 Tablespoons Ground Oatmeal~9.3g
5 3/4 cups Water

Healthy Method of Preparation:

- Combine meat, black pepper, flaxseed, and oatmeal in a large bowl
- Process in a blender with 1/2 cup of water until smooth paste is created
- Shape meat into balls
- In a deep cooking pan, place onions with 1 1/4 cups of water and bring to a boil over medium heat for 12 minutes, until water evaporates and onions are thick and juicy
- Add 4 cups of water and tomato paste; stir continuously for 2 minutes, until water is red
- Place meatballs in pan, cover and cook over medium heat, for another 20 minutes, until meat is brown
- Ready to serve

Nutritional Goal

The purpose of the modification is to reduce calories, to balance calories from macronutrients, to improve quality of fat, and to enrich food with fiber. The calorie content of the healthy recipe is reduced by more than 70% when compared to calorie content of the traditional recipe. In the healthy recipe, quality and quantity of fat are improved since total fat and saturated fat are reduced by more than 80%, and cholesterol is reduced by more than 45% when compared to their levels in the traditional recipe. Also, the reduction of omega-6-FA and the enrichment of omega-3-FA balance the ratio of these essential fatty acids in the healthy recipe. A comparison between the nutritional analysis of both recipes shows that fiber content of the healthy recipe is increased by more than 15%. The healthy recipe is recommended to individuals who like to consume meat but have high lipid profiles or heart disease.

Nutrient Content	Traditional Recipe	Healthy Recipe
Portion	1 cup	1 cup
Weight (g)	239	226
Kilocalories (kcal)	267.76	86.8
Protein (g)	11.4	6.9
Carbohydrate (g)	10	11.6
Fat (g)	20.8	2
Saturated Fat (g)	4.7	0.6
Monounsaturated Fat (g)	6.5	0.66
Polyunsaturated Fat (g)	7.8	0.6
Trans Fatty Acid (g)	0.5	0.1
Cholesterol (g)	35.3	14
Omega-6 Linoleic (g)	7.68	0.1
Omega-3 Linolenic (g)	0.12	0.34
Fiber (g)	2.02	2.4
Sugar (g)	5.19	4.7
Water (L)	0.1	0.4
Thiamin (mg)	0.1	0.1
Riboflavin (mg)	0.13	0.1
Niacin (mg)	3.4	2
Vitamin B6 (mg)	0.3	0.2
Vitamin B12 (mcg)	1.1	0.5
Folate (DFE) mcg	13.6	14
Vitamin C (mg)	9	7.9
Vitamin D (mcg)	0	0
Vitamin A (RAE) (mcg)	139.6	101
Vitamin E (mg)	3.3	0.88
Calcium (mg)	32.2	29
Iron (mg)	2.4	1.74
Magnesium (mg)	28.1	29
Potassium (mg)	525.5	400
Zinc (mg)	2.6	1.5
Sodium (mg)	273	188

Portion 1 Cup

Number of Exchanges

Traditional Recipe
1 2/3 meat exchange (medium fat)
1/3 non-starchy vegetable exchange
3 exchange of fat (PUFA)

Healthy Recipe
3/4 meat exchange (lean)
1/3 non-starchy vegetable exchange
2/3 fat exchange (Omega-3-FA)

Calories from Macronutrients

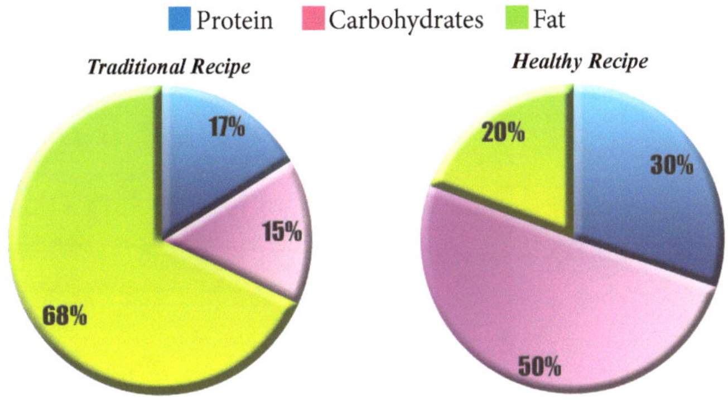

% Fiber Intake Compared to Average Daily Needs

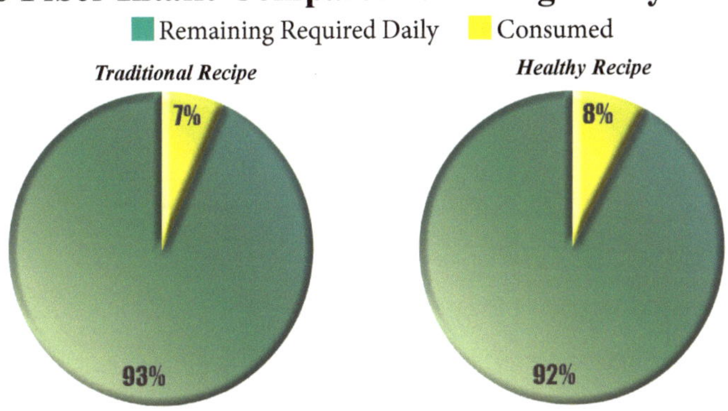

Recommended Portion Sizes & Meal Combinations

Traditional Recipe
(Calorie Controlled)

Men
1 1/2 cups of dawoud basha
3/4 cup of traditional egg noodle rice

Women
1 cup of dawoud basha
1/2 cup of traditional egg noodle rice

Healthy Recipe
(Calorie Controlled & Content Balanced)

Men
3 cups of dawoud basha
2/3 cup of healthy egg noodle rice
(see page:128)
3 cups of green salad-drizzled with olive oil & vinegar
1 cup of lowfat ayran

Women
1 1/4 cups of dawoud basha
1/2 cup of healthy egg noodle rice
(see page:128)
1 cup of green salad-drizzled with olive oil & vinegar
1 cup of lowfat ayran

Number of Exchanges in a Balanced Meal

Men
2 1/4 meat exchange (lean)
4 1/4 non-starchy vegetable exchange
2 1/2 grain exchange
1 milk exchange
4 1/4 fat exchange (1 3/4 Omega-3-FA,1 PUFA,1 1/2 MUFA)

Women
1 meat exchange (lean)
1 1/2 non-starchy vegetable exchange
2 grain exchange
1 milk exchange
2 fat exchange (3/4 Omega-3-FA, 3/4 PUFA, 1/2 MUFA)

Meat Rolls Grilled with Tomatoes & Onions

(Kabbab Bel Al Tamatum)

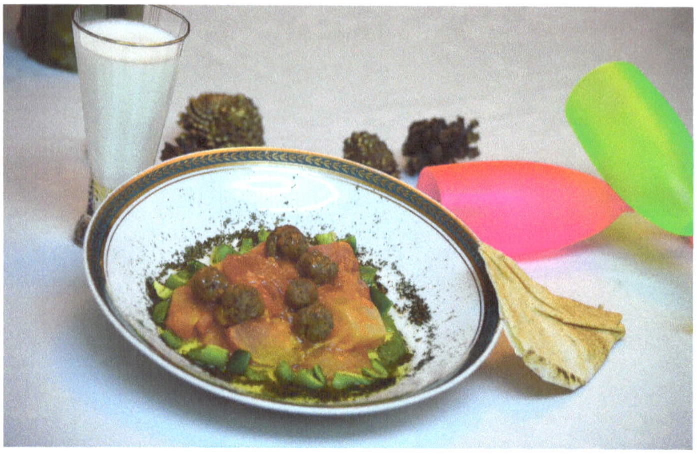

Traditional Recipe, 4 Servings, 4 Cups:

12 oz. Medium Fat Ground Meat~342g
4 2/3 cups Peeled Diced Tomatoes~1122g
1/2 cup Chopped Onions~88g
2 teaspoons Black Pepper~4g
1/4 cup Water

Traditional Method of Preparation:

- Wash tomatoes carefully, soak in hot water for 3 minutes, until they are easy to peel
- Cut peeled tomatoes into quarters
- Combine meat, black pepper, and onion in a large bowl
- Add 1/4 cup of water; the mixture should be moist but easy to hold its shape if rolled
- Shape into finger-sized links or small balls
- Pre-heat the oven at high heat for 10 minutes
- In an oven dish, place diced tomatoes on base and arrange meat
- Roast in moderately heated oven for 40 minutes
- Ready to serve

Healthy Recipe, 4 Servings, 4 Cups:

8 oz. Lean Meat~229.56g
4 1/4 cups Peeled Diced Tomatoes~1033.02g
1 1/2 cup Chopped Onions~229.56g
4 teaspoons Black pepper~8g
3 3/4 Tablespoons Ground Oatmeal~22.9g
3 3/4 Tablespoons Ground Flaxseed~28.6g
4 teaspoons Sumac powder
5 cups Water

Healthy Method of Preparation:

- Wash tomatoes carefully, soak in warm water for 3 minutes, until they are easy to peel
- Cut peeled tomatoes into quarters
- Combine meat, black pepper, oatmeal, sumac and onions in a large bowl
- Process mixture in a blender and add 2 cups of water, until it forms a smooth paste
- Add 1 cup of water to mixture; the mixture should be moist but easy to hold its shape if rolled
- Shape into finger-sized links or small balls
- Pre-heat the oven at high heat for 10 minutes
- In an oven dish, place diced tomatoes on base and arrange meats
- Roast in moderately heated oven, for 40 minutes. Add 2 cups of water every 10 minutes
- Sprinkle flaxseed over food
- Ready to serve

  *Optional: combine flaxseed with meat mixture before blending

Nutritional Goal

The modification of this recipe results in great nutritional outcomes. The quality and quantity of fat are significantly improved in the healthy recipe. Total fat and saturated fat are reduced by more than 70%, when omega 3-fatty acid is increased by more than 1000%. The change in fat content balances the calories from macronutrients in the healthy recipe. The calorie content of the healthy recipe is reduced by more than 35% when compared to calorie content of the traditional recipe. The fiber content of the healthy recipe is also increased by more 65% when compared to fiber content of the traditional recipe. In addition, the healthy recipe contains more niacin, folate, calcium, magnesium, zinc, and potassium, according to the result of the nutritional analysis. The healthy recipe is highly recommended to athletes, children, individuals who like to eat meat, and individuals with excessive body weight and malnutrition.

Nutrient Content	Traditional Recipe	Healthy Recipe
Portion	1 cup	1 cup
Weight (g)	241	264
Kilocalories (kcal)	346.3	206.7
Protein (g)	15.1	17.1
Carbohydrate (g)	13.9	22
Fat (g)	26.26	6.6
Saturated Fat (g)	9.8	1.7
Monounsaturated Fat (g)	11.4	1.9
Polyunsaturated Fat (g)	0.99	2.7
Trans Fatty Acid (g)	1.56	0.2
Cholesterol (g)	66.7	35.6
Omega-6 Linoleic (g)	0.87	0.44
Omega-3 Linolenic (g)	0.1	1.7
Fiber (g)	3.8	6.5
Sugar (g)	8.3	9.6
Water (L)	0.33	1.5
Thiamin (mg)	0.15	0.28
Riboflavin (mg)	0.18	0.17
Niacin (mg)	4.6	5.2
Vitamin B6 (mg)	0.5	0.6
Vitamin B12 (mcg)	1.77	1.3
Folate (DFE) mcg	53.1	60
Vitamin C (mg)	37.3	36.5
Vitamin D (mcg)	0	0
Vitamin A (RAE) (mcg)	708.7	652
Vitamin E (mg)	0.9	0.97
Calcium (mg)	58	63.9
Iron (mg)	2.5	2.8
Magnesium (mg)	47.1	81.5
Potassium (mg)	896.3	975.2
Zinc (mg)	3.6	3.9
Sodium (mg)	72	54.9

Portion 1 Cup

Number of Exchanges

Traditional Recipe
2 3/4 meat exchange (medium fat)
1 1/3 non-starchy vegetable exchange

Healthy Recipe
2 meat exchange (lean)
1 1/2 non-starchy vegetable exchange
1/3 grain exchange
3 fat exchange (Omega-3-FA)

Calories from Macronutrients

Protein Carbohydrates Fat

Traditional Recipe

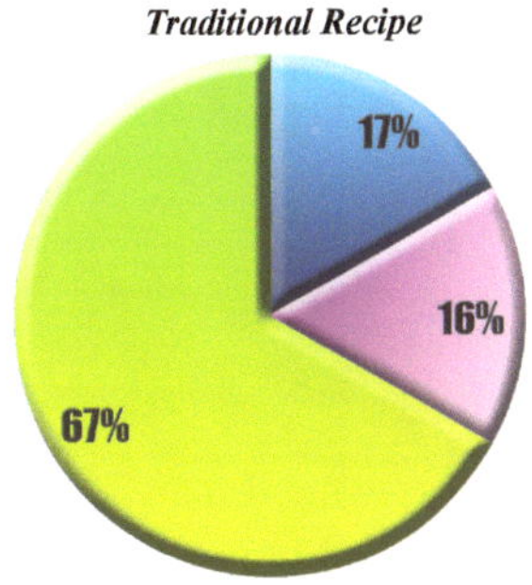

Healthy Recipe

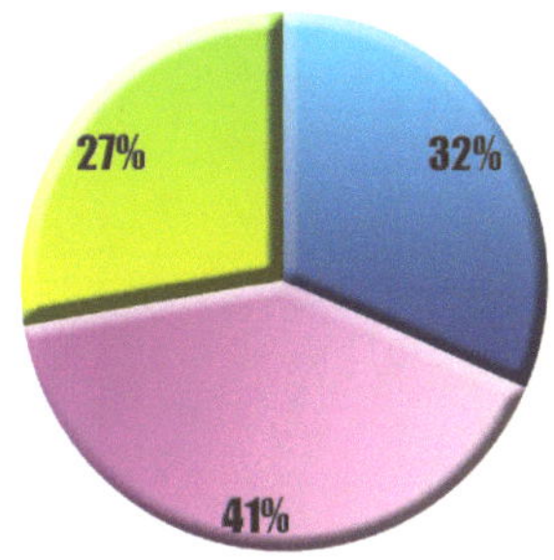

% Fiber Intake Compared to Average Daily Needs

Remaining Required Daily Consumed

Traditional Recipe

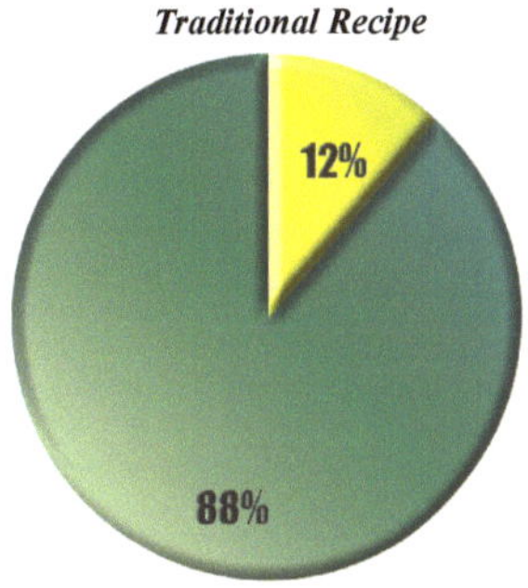

Healthy Recipe

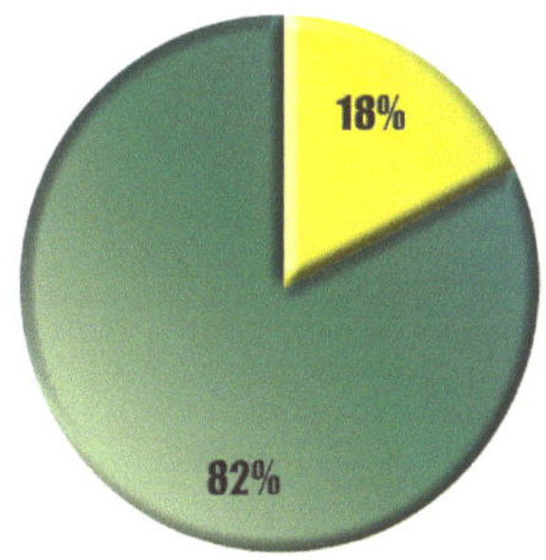

Recommended Portion Sizes & Meal Combinations

Traditional Recipe
(Calorie Controlled)

Men
1 3/4 cups of kabbab bel al tamatum
2 slices of small white pita bread

Women
1 1/4 cups kabbab bel al tamatum
3/4 slice of small white pita bread

Healthy Recipe
(Calorie Controlled & Content Balanced)

Men
2 1/4 cups of kabbab bel al tamatum
2 slices of small whole wheat pita bread
2 cups of green salad-drizzled with vinegar
1 cup of lowfat ayran

Women
1 1/2 cups of kabbab bel al tamatum
1 slice of small whole wheat pita bread
1 cup of green salad-drizzled with vinegar
1 cup of lowfat ayran

Number of Exchanges in a Balanced Meal

Men
4 meat exchange (lean)
5 1/3 non-starchy vegetable exchange
2 2/3 grain exchange
6 1/3 fat exchange (Omega-3-FA)
1 milk exchange

Women
2 3/4 meat exchange (lean)
3 non-starchy vegetable exchange
1 1/2 grain exchange
4 1/4 fat exchange (Omega-3-FA)
1 milk exchange

Oven-Grilled Meat

(Lahem Be Al-Fouron)

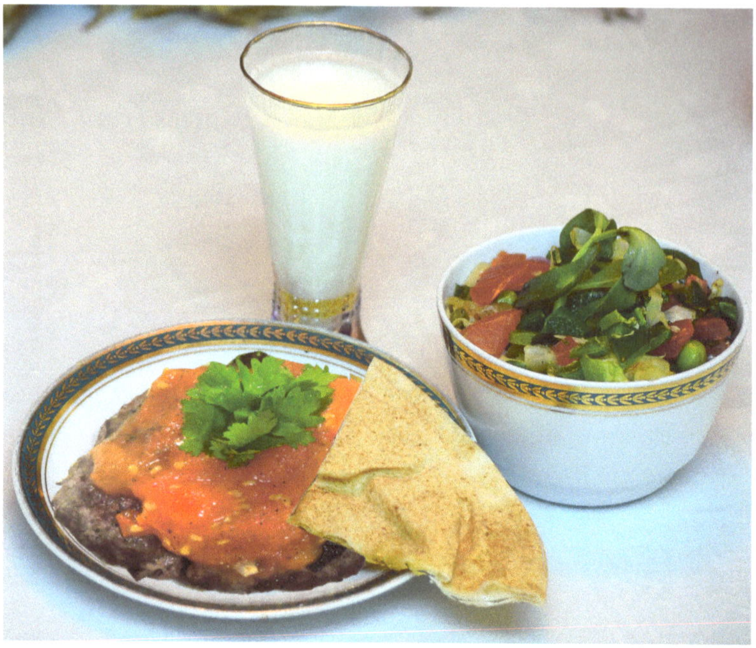

Traditional Recipe, 4 Servings, 4 Cups:

12 oz. Medium Fat Ground Meat~339.76g
1/2 cup Chopped Onions~83.29g
1/4 cup Sliced Tomatoes~67.95g
4 1/3 Tablespoons Pomegranate Molasses~71.89g
2 teaspoons Black Pepper~4g

Healthy Recipe, 4 Servings, 4 Cups:

12.5 oz. Lean Meat~353g
3/4 cup Chopped Onions~116g
2 1/3 cups Sliced Tomatoes~ 564.928g
3 Tablespoons Pomegranate Molasses~48.56g
3 Tablespoons Ground Flaxseed~22.06g
6 Tablespoons Ground Oatmeal~35.3g
9 cups Water

Traditional Method of Preparation:

- Combine meat, black pepper, onions, and pomegranate molasses in a large bowl
- Process in a blender and spread in an oven dish
- Pre-heat oven at high heat for 10 minutes
- Decorate meat with tomato slices
- Roast in medium high heated oven for 45 minutes until meat is brown
- Ready to serve

Healthy Method of Preparation:

- Combine meat, black pepper, oatmeal, flaxseed and onions in a large bowl
- Process in a blender; blending mixture until it is smooth paste
- Pre-heat oven at high heat for 10 minutes
- Place meat in an oven dish and cover meat with tomato slices
- Roast in moderately heated oven for 45 minutes
  Add 3 1/2 cups of water every 20 minutes
- Ready to serve

Nutritional Goal

The modification of this recipe is highly recommended since it greatly improves the nutritional values of the food. Calories of the healthy recipe are reduced by more than 70%, when compared to calories of the traditional recipe. Fat quality is improved in the healthy recipe; trans fatty acid is nearly eliminated, saturated fat and cholesterol are reduced by more than 70%, and omega-3-FA is increased by more than 300%. The increase of omega-3-FA balances the ratio of omega-6: omega-3 of the healthy recipe when compared to the ratio of omega-6: omega-3 in the traditional recipe. Fiber is also enriched with more than 130% in the healthy recipe when compared to fiber content of the traditional recipe. The healthy recipe is recommended to athletes, children, dieters, and individuals who over consume meat.

Nutrient Content	Traditional Recipe	Healthy Recipe
Portion	1 cup	1 cup
Weight (g)	85	84.992
Kilocalories (kcal)	354.6	78.3188
Protein (g)	14.4	7.5364
Carbohydrate (g)	11	6.972
Fat (g)	28	2.324
Saturated Fat (g)	10.5	0.7636
Monounsaturated Fat (g)	12.3	0.83
Polyunsaturated Fat (g)	0.74	0.664
Trans Fatty Acid (g)	78	0.0996
Cholesterol (g)	72.7	18.1604
Omega-6 Linoleic (g)	0.6	0.12284
Omega-3 Linolenic (g)	0.1	0.4316
Fiber (g)	1	1.5936
Sugar (g)	8	3.2204
Water (L)	0.12	0.5312
Thiamin (mg)	0.1	0.07636
Riboflavin (mg)	0.16	0.0664
Niacin (mg)	3.4	2.0916
Vitamin B6 (mg)	0.4	0.1992
Vitamin B12 (mcg)	1.9	0.664
Folate (DFE) mcg	16.4	13.2136
Vitamin C (mg)	6.4	7.138
Vitamin D (mcg)	0	0
Vitamin A (RAE) (mcg)	57	121.3792
Vitamin E (mg)	0.3	0.2324
Calcium (mg)	40	15.3716
Iron (mg)	2.4	1.0624
Magnesium (mg)	23	23.3728
Potassium (mg)	407	276.556
Zinc (mg)	3.5	1.7596
Sodium (mg)	66	22.8748

Portion:3 oz (85g)

Number of Exchanges

Traditional Recipe

2 3/4 meat exchange (medium fat)

Healthy Recipe

3 meat exchange (lean)
3/4 non-starchy vegetable exchange
2 1/4 fat exchange (Omega-3-FA)
1/2 grain exchange

Calories from Macronutrients

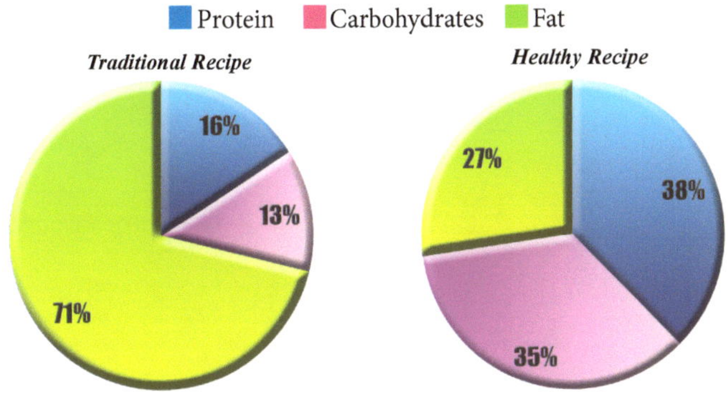

% Fiber Intake Compared to Average Daily Needs

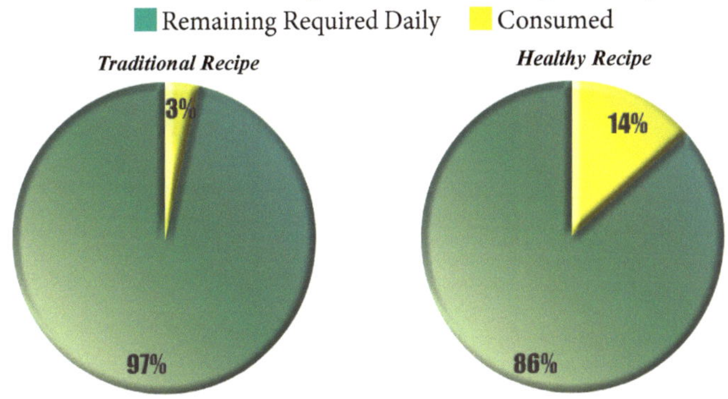

Recommended Portion Sizes & Meal Combinations

Traditional Recipe
(Calorie Controlled)

Men
1 3/4 serving of lahem be Al-fouron
2 slices of small white pita bread

Women
1 serving of lahem be Al-fouron
1 1/2 slices of small white pita bread

Healthy Recipe
(Calorie Controlled & Content Balanced)

Men
1 1/2 serving of lahem be Al-fouron
2 slices of small white pita bread
2 cups of green salad-drizzled with olive oil
1 cup of lowfat ayran

Women
1 serving of lahem be Al-fouron
1 slice of small white pita bread
1 cup of green salad-drizzled with olive oil
1 cup of lowfat ayran

Number of Exchanges in a Balanced Meal

Men
4 1/4 meat exchange (lean)
3 non-starchy vegetable exchange
5 1/3 fat exchange
(2 MUFA, 3 1/3 Omega-3-FA)
2 3/4 grain exchange
1 milk exchange

Women
3 meat exchange (lean)
1 3/4 non-starchy vegetable exchange
3 1/4 fat exchange
(1 MUFA, 2 1/4 Omega-3-FA)
1 1/2 grain exchange
1 milk exchange

Dairy

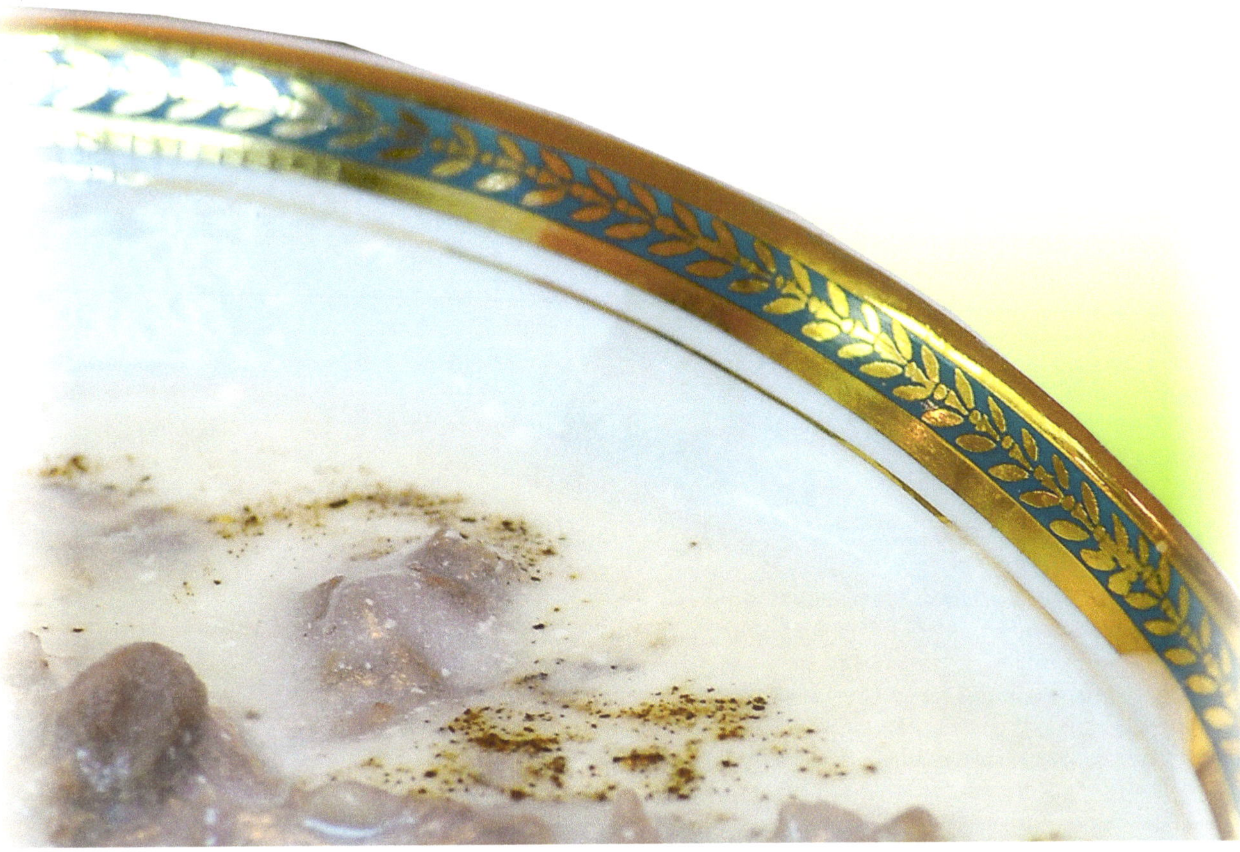

Eggplant Paste

(Motabal Bazenjan)

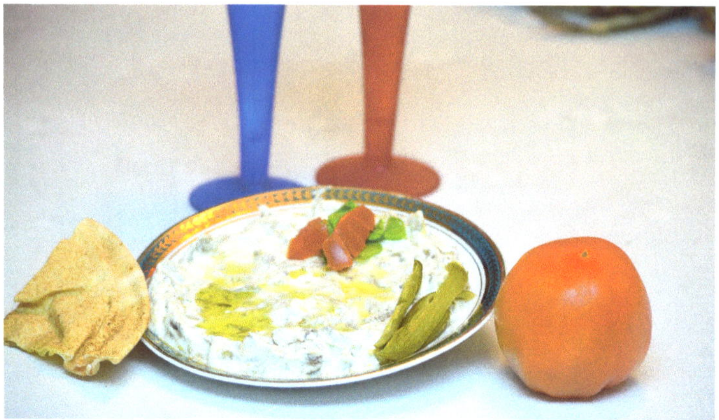

Traditional Recipe, 4 Servings, 4 Cups:

5 cups Eggplant~713.4g
5 Tablespoons Ground Garlic~61.5g
1 1/4 cups Regular Yogurt~320g
1 cup Lemon Juice~270.6g
3 1/3 Tablespoons Tahini~ 49.2g
6 1/3 Tablespoons Corn Oil~ 86.1g
Optional: Olive Oil and Parsley for decoration

Healthy Recipe, 4 Servings, 4 Cups:

7 1/2 cups Eggplant~1066g
7 2/3 Tablespoons Ground Garlic~92g
2 cups Lowfat Yogurt~477.88g
1 2/3 cups Lemon Juice~ 404.36g
5 Tablespoons Tahini~73.52g
Optional: Olive Oil and Parsley for decoration

Traditional Method of Preparation:

- Remove green stem and wash eggplant gently
- Peel off skin; slice into thick pieces
- Heat oil and deep fry eggplant over high heat for 5 minutes, turning often until eggplant is golden brown
- Chop eggplant in mortar to puree or process in food blender
- Place ground garlic with eggplant and continue chopping until the mixture is homogenous
- In a large bowl, combine all the ingredients together, stir rapidly using a large fork
- Place mixture in shallow dish; drizzle with parsley and olive oil
- Ready to serve as an appetizer

Healthy Method of Preparation:

- Wash eggplant carefully; leave stem for convenient handling
- Lay the eggplants on the rock oven, and grill in hot oven for 20 minutes until tender, turning frequently
- While hot, peel off skin and remove stem
- Chop eggplant in mortar to puree or process in food blender
- Place ground garlic with eggplant and continue chopping until the mixture homogenous
- In a large bowl, combine all ingredients together, stir at high speed using large fork
- Place in shallow dish; drizzle with parsley and 4 teaspoons of olive oil
- Ready to serve as an appetizer

Nutritional Goal

The modification of this food is essential. The traditional recipe is nutritionally poor due to multiple features such as high calorie content, high level of bad fat, low fiber content, and low contents of carbohydrate and protein. The calorie content of the healthy recipe is reduced by more than 60%, when compared to the traditional recipe. In the healthy recipe, the total fat is also reduced by more than 70%, when carbohydrate and protein are increased by more than 30% resulting in more balanced proportion of macronutrients. Also, the omega-6: omega-3 value is healthier in the healthy recipe, 3:1, in contrast to 78:1 in the traditional recipe. The fiber content of healthy recipe is also increased by more than 40%, when compared to fiber content of the traditional recipe. A comparison between nutritional analysis of the recipes shows that the healthy recipe contains higher levels of thiamin, riboflavin, niacin, vitamin B6, vitamin B12, folate, vitamin C, vitamin A, calcium, iron, magnesium, potassium, and zinc. The healthy recipe is recommended to individuals with digestive problems and heart disease.

Nutrient Content	Traditional Recipe	Healthy Recipe
Portion	1 cup	1 cup
Weight (g)	261.375	312.46
Kilocalories (kcal)	1086.8	331.3
Protein (g)	10.2	15.3
Carbohydrate (g)	27.7	39.3
Fat (g)	107.4	15
Saturated Fat (g)	14.9	4
Monounsaturated Fat (g)	24.26	1.03
Polyunsaturated Fat (g)	57.5	0.35
Trans Fatty Acid (g)	0.28	0
Cholesterol (g)	7.7	12.4
Omega-6 Linoleic (g)	56.8	0.28
Omega-3 Linolenic (g)	0.73	0.1
Fiber (g)	7.9	11.7
Sugar (g)	10	15
Water (L)	0.3	0.45
Thiamin (mg)	0.16	0.24
Riboflavin (mg)	0.27	0.4
Niacin (mg)	1.4	2
Vitamin B6 (mg)	0.42	0.6
Vitamin B12 (mcg)	0.45	0.7
Folate (DFE) mcg	48.5	70.5
Vitamin C (mg)	40.3	52
Vitamin D (mcg)	0	0
Vitamin A (RAE) (mcg)	38	58
Vitamin E (mg)	17	0.22
Calcium (mg)	194	295.8
Iron (mg)	1.4	1.9
Magnesium (mg)	45	67
Potassium (mg)	737.6	1088
Zinc (mg)	1	1.7
Sodium (mg)	60	94

Portion 1 Cup

Number of Exchanges

Traditional Recipe
1/2 milk exchange
6 fat exchange
(1 1/4 MUFA, 4 3/4 PUFA)
1 1/4 non-starchy vegetable exchange

Healthy Recipe
3/4 milk exchange
2 fat exchange (MUFA)
2 non-starchy vegetable exchange

Calories from Macronutrients

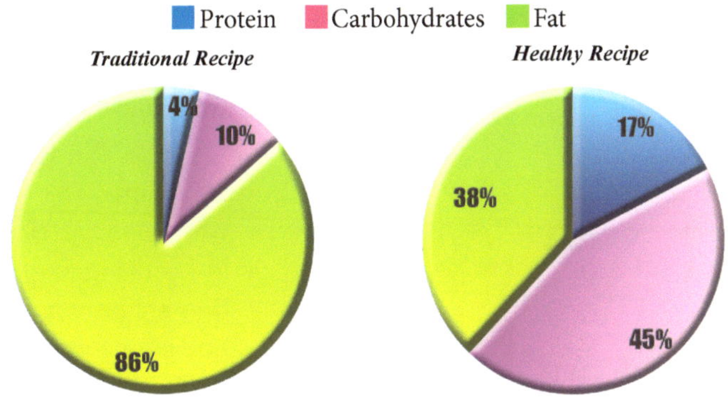

% Fiber Intake Compared to Average Daily Needs

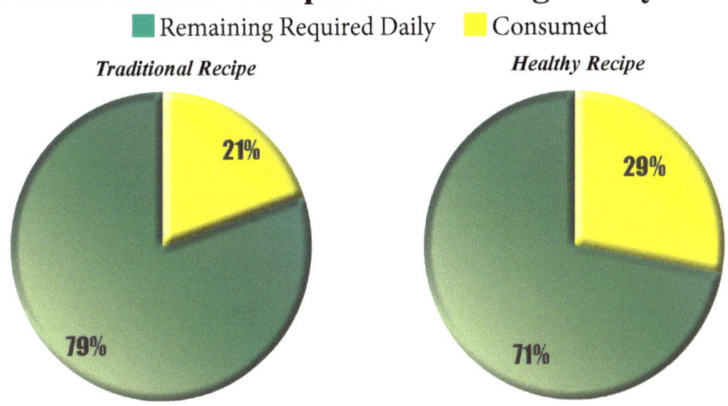

Recommended Portion Sizes & Meal Combinations

Traditional Recipe
(Calorie Controlled)

Men
1/4 cup of motabal bazenjan
3/4 slice of small white pita bread

Women
2 1/2 tablespoons motabal bazenjan
1/3 slice of small white pita bread

Healthy Recipe
(Calorie Controlled & Content Balanced)

Men
3/4 cup of motabal bazenjan
3/4 slice of small white pita bread

Women
1/2 cup of motabal bazenjan
1/2 slice of small white pita bread

Number of Exchanges in a Balanced Meal

Men
2/3 milk exchange
1 1/3 fat exchange (MUFA)
1 1/3 non-starchy vegetable exchange
3/4 grain exchange

Women
1/3 milk exchange
1 fat exchange (MUFA)
1 non-starchy vegetable exchange
1/2 grain exchange

Okra Stewed with Meat & Yogurt
(Makhtoum Bamyah)

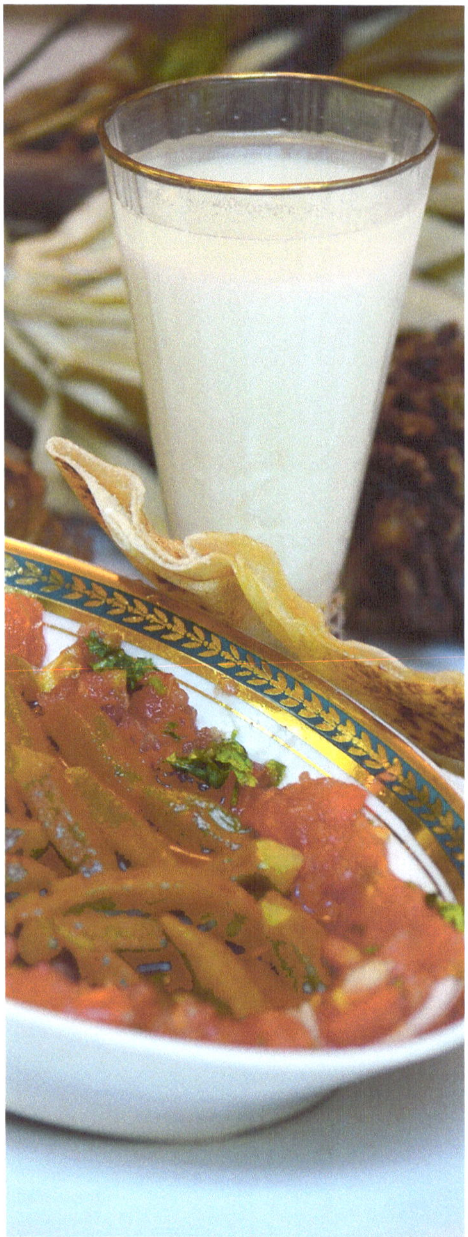

Traditional Recipe, 4 Servings, 4 Cups:

8.2 oz. Cooked Shank Meat~232g
1 Tablespoon Chopped Onions~15.5g
3 1/4 cups Raw Okra~324.2g
1 cup Lemon Juice~235g
1 cup Chopped Tomatoes~288g
1/3 cup Regular Yogurt~105g
1 Tablespoon Corn Oil~15g
2 2/3 teaspoons Cardamom Ground~6.5g
2 2/3 teaspoons Cinnamon Ground~6.5g
10 cups Water

Traditional Method of Preparation:

- In a large pan, place meat with 10 cups of water and cook over medium heat for 20 minutes
- Wash okra and drain
- In a cooking pan, heat oil and fry onions over medium heat for 3 minutes until they are brown
- Add okra, tomatoes, cardamom, and cinnamon to onions; cover and cook over medium heat for 5 minutes; stir frequently
- Combine meat and meat stock with cooked vegetables
- Add lemon juice and yogurt and continue to cook over medium heat for another 20 minutes; stir frequently
- Ready to serve

Healthy Recipe, 4 Servings, 4 Cups:

2.5 oz. Lean Meat~69g
1/2 cup Chopped Onions~83.44g
2 3/4 cups Steamed Okra~495g
3/4 cup Lemon Juice~180g
1 1/3 cups Chopped Tomatoes~333.7g
1/2 cup Lowfat Yogurt~113.5g
2 Tablespoons Tomato Juice~55.7g
2 3/4 teaspoons Ground Cardamom~7g
2 3/4 teaspoons Ground Cinnamon~7g
4 1/2 cups Water

Healthy Method of Preparation:

- In a large pan, combine meat and onions with 4 1/2 cups of water; cook over medium heat for 20 minutes
- Wash okra and steam at high heat for 15 minutes
- Add steamed okra, tomatoes, tomato juice, cardamom, and cinnamon
- Cover and continue to cook over medium heat for another 5 minutes; stirring frequently
- Add lemon juice and yogurt and continue to cook over medium heat for additional 20 minutes; stir frequently
- Ready to serve

Nutritional Goal

The modification aims to reduce calories, to control quality and quantity of fat, and to enrich food with fiber and nutrients. The calorie content of the healthy recipe is reduced by more than 30%, when compared to the calorie content of the traditional recipe. The quantity and quality of fat are controlled in the healthy recipe; trans fatty acid is eliminated. Total fat, saturated fat, and cholesterol are reduced by more than 75% in the healthy recipe when compared to their levels in the traditional recipe. The reduction of animal-based protein, meat, along with the addition of complex carbohydrate, and okra result in much healthier proportion of macronutrients, as calories from the macronutrient charts show. This change also leads to an increase in fiber content in the healthy recipe. A comparison between nutritional analysis of both recipes show that both recipes are nutrient condensed; however, the healthy recipe contains higher levels of folate, calcium, and magnesium. The healthy recipe is recommended to postmenopausal women, folate deficiency anemia, athletes, and individuals with high lipid profiles and excessive body weight.

Nutrient Content	Traditional Recipe	Healthy Recipe
Portion	1 cup	1 cup
Weight (g)	220	220
Kilocalories (kcal)	235.5	124.9
Protein (g)	13.3	7.9
Carbohydrate (g)	18.9	23.3
Fat (g)	13.5	2
Saturated Fat (g)	5.3	0.8
Monounsaturated Fat (g)	4.4	0.6
Polyunsaturated Fat (g)	2.8	0.3
Trans Fatty Acid (g)	0.01	0
Cholesterol (g)	39.5	8
Omega-6 Linoleic (g)	2.5	0.2
Omega-3 Linolenic (g)	0.2	0.02
Fiber (g)	4.7	6
Sugar (g)	7.3	9.6
Water (L)	0.4	23.4
Thiamin (mg)	0.2	0.2
Riboflavin (mg)	0.4	0.26
Niacin (mg)	4.4	2.3
Vitamin B6 (mg)	0.2	0.3
Vitamin B12 (mcg)	1.5	0.6
Folate (DFE) mcg	139.7	200.7
Vitamin C (mg)	46.6	50
Vitamin D (mcg)	0	0
Vitamin A (RAE) (mcg)	277.7	348.6
Vitamin E (mg)	1.5	1.1
Calcium (mg)	154	191.8
Iron (mg)	2.05	2
Magnesium (mg)	66.8	81.3
Potassium (mg)	590.5	726
Zinc (mg)	2.8	2.3
Sodium (mg)	47	73

Portion 1 Cup

Number of Exchanges

Traditional Recipe
2 meat exchange (high fat)
1 non-starchy vegetable exchange
3/4 fat exchange (PUFA)

Healthy Recipe
1/2 meat exchange (medium fat)
2 non-starchy vegetable exchange

Calories from Macronutrients

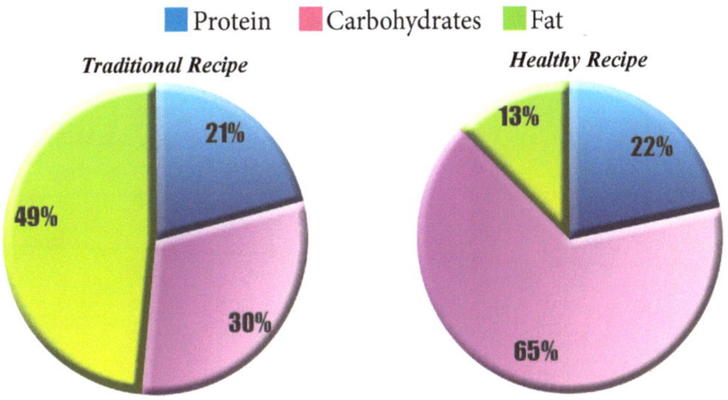

% Fiber Intake Compared to Average Daily Needs

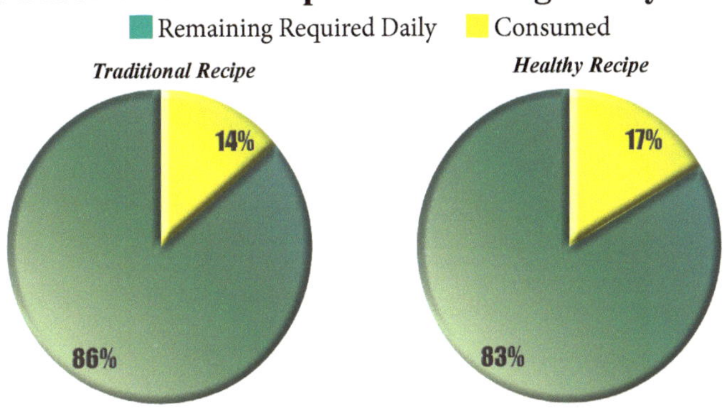

Recommended Portion Sizes & Meal Combinations

Traditional Recipe
(Calorie Controlled)

Men
2 1/2 cups of makhtoum bamyah
2 1/2 slices of small white pita bread

Women
1 1/2 cups of makhtoum bamyah
1 1/2 slices of small white pita bread

Healthy Recipe
(Calorie Controlled & Content Balanced)

Men
4 cups of makhtoum bamyah
3 slices of small whole wheat pita bread
1/2 cup lowfat ayran

Women
2 1/2 cups of makhtoum bamyah
1 1/4 slices of small whole wheat pita bread
1 cup lowfat ayran

Number of Exchanges in a Balanced Meal

Men
2 meat exchange (medium fat)
7 1/2 non-starchy vegetable exchange
1 1/3 milk exchange
3 grain exchange

Women
1 1/4 meat exchange (medium fat)
4 3/4 non-starchy vegetable exchange
1 1/2 milk exchange
1 1/4 grain exchange

Shank Meat Cooked in Yogurt

(Shakreyah)

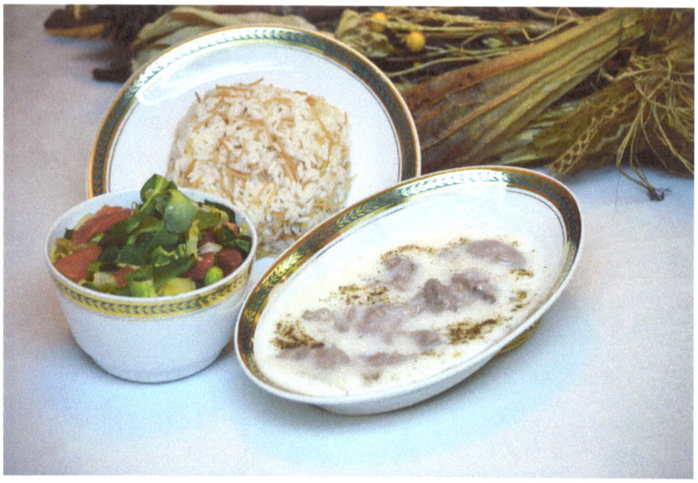

Traditional Recipe, 4 Servings, 4 Cups:

4 1/4 Tablespoons Starch~34g
3 1/2 cups Regular Plain Yogurt~838g
1 Medium Egg~46g
11 oz. Shank Meat~316 g
3/4 cup Sliced Onions~120g
18 cups Water

Traditional Method of Preparation:

- In a cooking pan, bring 18 cups of water to boil and cook shank meat with sliced onions over medium heat for 30 minutes until meat is tender
- In another cooking pan, place yogurt over medium heat and stir until yogurt begins to simmer
- Sprinkle in starch and stir until yogurt thickens
- Beat an egg and stir into mixture until it is dissolved thoroughly
- Transfer meat, and sliced onions to yogurt mixture
- Cook for another 20 minutes over medium heat until mixture is homogenous
- Ready to serve

Healthy Recipe, 4 Servings, 4 Cups:

1 Tablespoon Starch~9g
2 2/3 cups Lowfat Plain Yogurt~ 644g
2.6 oz. Lean Shank Meat~74g
1 1/3 cups Chopped Onions~ 216g
2 teaspoons Ground Flaxseed~ 5.25g
8 cups Water

Healthy Method of Preparation:

- In a cooking pan, bring 8 cups of water to boil and cook shank meat with sliced onions over medium heat for 25 minutes until meat is tender and brown
- In another cooking pan, place yogurt over medium heat and stir until yogurt begins to simmer
- Sprinkle in starch and stir until yogurt thickens
- Transfer meat broth, meat, and sliced onions to yogurt mixture
- Cook for another 20 minutes over medium heat until mixture is homogenous
- Add flaxseed; stir twice
- Ready to serve

Nutritional Goal

The purpose of the modification is to reduce calories, to balance proportion of macronutrients, and to enrich food with fiber. The changes in the ratio of onions, meat, and by omitting egg in the method of yogurt preparation, are the main reasons for the great nutritional values of the healthy recipe. This recipe has multiple nutritional benefits when compared to the traditional recipe. Calorie content of the healthy recipe is reduced by more than half. Total fat, saturated fat, and cholesterol are greatly reduced by more than 60%. Thus, macronutrient contents are much more balanced, and fat is no longer predominant. Fiber content of the healthy recipe is as twice as fiber content of the traditional recipe. Also, sodium content of the healthy recipe is reduced by more than 25% when compared to sodium content of the traditional recipe. This food is recommended to individuals who enjoy eating meat but having a chronic illness such as heart disease, high lipid profiles, high blood pressure, digestive problems, and obesity.

Nutrient Content	Traditional Recipe	Healthy Recipe
Portion	1 cup	1 cup
Weight (g)	333.5	240
Kilocalories (kcal)	385	171
Protein (g)	26	11.5
Carbohydrate (g)	25	19
Fat (g)	20	6
Saturated Fat (g)	10.5	3
Monounsaturated Fat (g)	7	1.6
Polyunsaturated Fat (g)	1	0.6
Trans Fatty Acid (g)	0	0
Cholesterol (g)	62	21
Omega-6 Linoleic (g)	0.56	0.1
Omega-3 Linolenic (g)	0.3	0.34
Fiber (g)	0.5	1
Sugar (g)	12	11
Water (L)	0.3	11
Thiamin (mg)	0.24	0.15
Riboflavin (mg)	1	0.4
Niacin (mg)	5	1
Vitamin B6 (mg)	0.3	0.2
Vitamin B12 (mcg)	3.3	1.4
Folate (DFE) mcg	12	13
Vitamin C (mg)	3	4.3
Vitamin D (mcg)	0.15	0
Vitamin A (RAE) (mcg)	67	39
Vitamin E (mg)	0.24	0.25
Calcium (mg)	355	277.4
Iron (mg)	1.6	0.6
Magnesium (mg)	49	38
Potassium (mg)	634	511
Zinc (mg)	4.4	2.4
Sodium (mg)	180	110

Portion 1 Cup

Number of Exchanges

Traditional Recipe
1 1/2 milk exchange
1/3 grain exchange
2 3/4 meat exchange (2 1/2 high fat, 1/4 medium fat and substitute)

Healthy Recipe
1 milk exchange
1/2 fat exchange (Omega-3-FA)
1/3 non-starchy vegetable exchange
2/3 meat exchange (lean)

Calories from Macronutrients

Protein Carbohydrates Fat

Traditional Recipe   *Healthy Recipe*

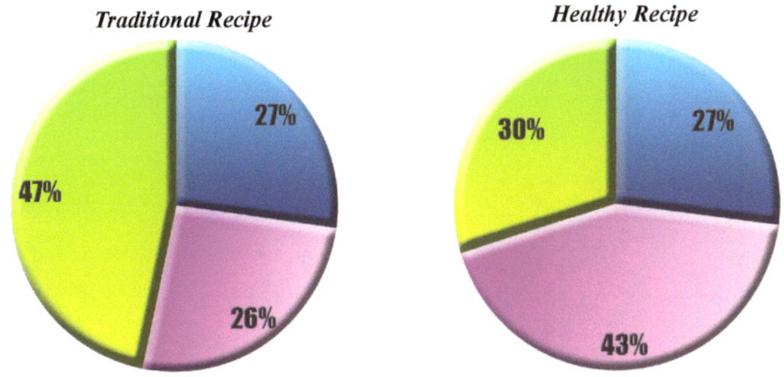

% Fiber Intake Compared to Average Daily Needs

Remaining Required Daily Consumed

Traditional Recipe   *Healthy Recipe*

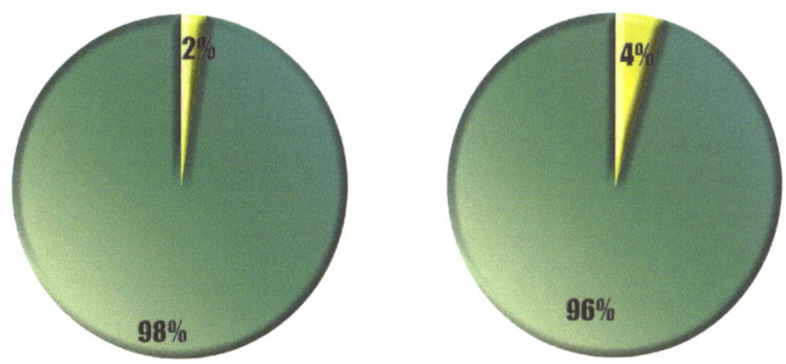

Recommended Portion Sizes & Meal Combinations

Traditional Recipe
(Calorie Controlled)

Men
1 cup of shakreyah
3/4 cup of traditional egg noodle rice

Women
3/4 cup of shakreyah
1/3 cup of traditional egg noodle rice

Healthy Recipe
(Calorie Controlled & Content Balanced)

Men
2 cups of shakreyah
3/4 cup of healthy egg noodle rice (see page:128)
3 cups of green salad-drizzled with vinegar

Women
1 1/4 cups of shakreyah
1/2 cup of healthy egg noodle rice (see page:128)
1 3/4 cups of green salad-drizzled with vinegar

Number of Exchanges in a Balanced Meal

Men
1 meat exchange (lean)
3 2/3 non-starchy vegetable exchange
2 fat exchange (1 PUFA, 1 Omega-3-FA)
2 milk exchange
3 grain exchange

Women
3/4 meat exchange (lean)
2 non-starchy vegetable exchange
1 1/3 fat exchange (3/4 PUFA, 2/3 Omega-3-FA)
1 1/4 milk exchange
2 grain exchange

VEGETABLES

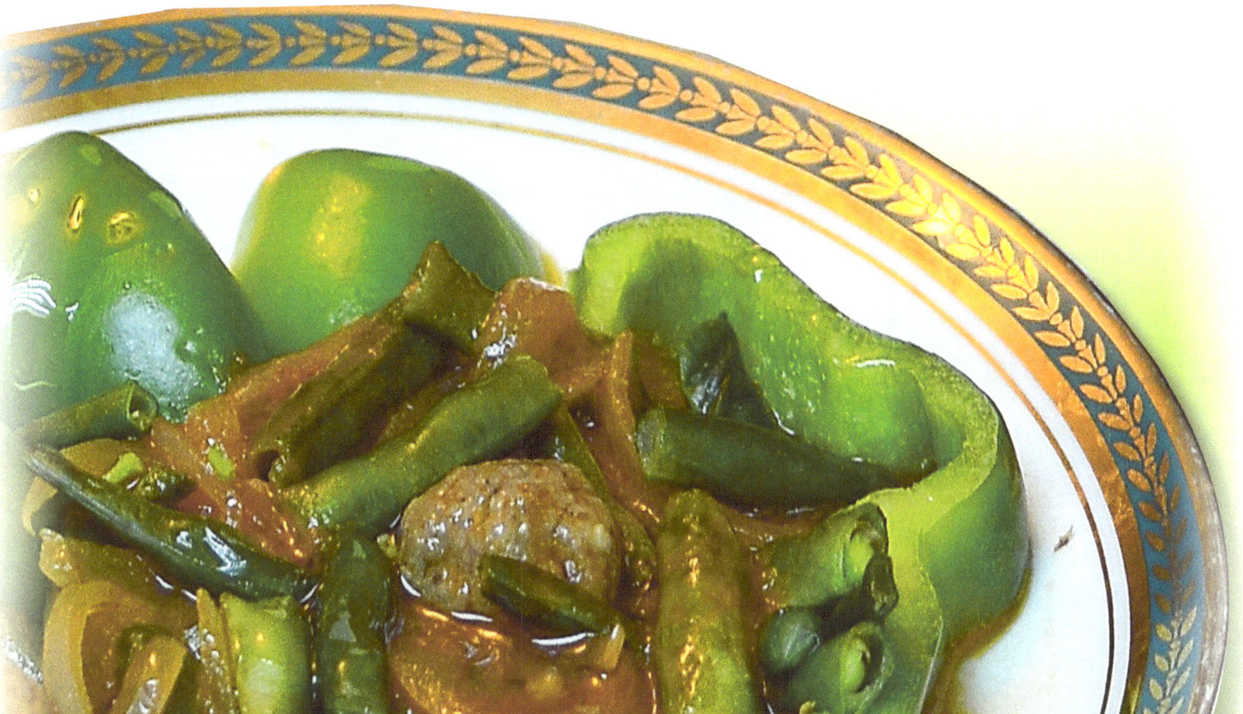

Cauliflower Stewed with Meat & Cilantro
(Qarnabit Monazal)

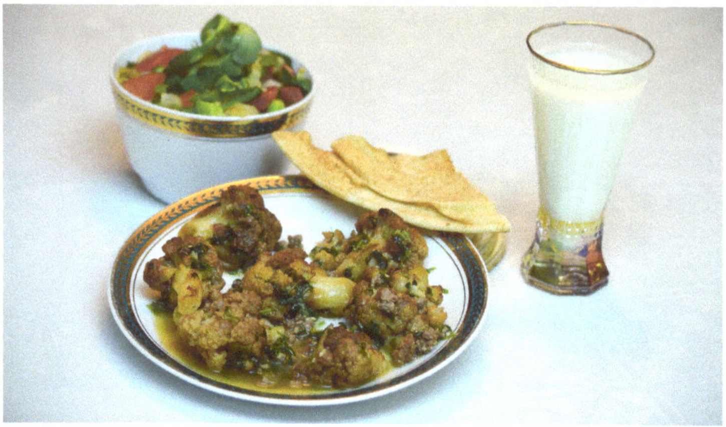

Traditional Recipe, 4 Servings, 4 Cups:

1 2/3 cups Chopped Cauliflower~316g
15 oz. Ground Meat~428g
1/3 cup Chopped Onions~68g
3 1/2 Tablespoons Fresh Cilantro~45g
1 teaspoon Black Pepper~2g
7 1/2 Tablespoons Corn Oil~101.5g
10 cups Water

Traditional Method of Preparation:

- Season meat with black pepper
- Wash, drain, and chop cauliflower
- In a cooking pan, heat oil and fry onions over medium heat for 5 minutes
- Combine meat with onions; continue cooking for 10 minutes until meat is tender
- Add cauliflower and continue to cooking; stir frequently for 5 minutes
- Add 10 cups of water and cook over medium heat for 30 minutes until cauliflower is tender; stir occasionally
- Reduce heat, add cilantro; cover and cook over low heat for 5 minutes
- Ready to serve

Healthy Recipe, 4 Servings, 4 Cups:

2 1/3 cups Chopped Cauliflower~446g
2.8 oz. Lean Ground Meat~80.3g
3/4 cup Chopped Onions~134g
1/2 cup Fresh Cilantro~104g
1 teaspoon Black pepper~2g
4 Tablespoons Ground Flaxseed~30g
4 cups Lemon Juice~954.5g
5 3/4 cups Water

Healthy Method of Preparation:

- Season meat with black pepper
- Wash, drain, and chop cauliflower
- In a cooking pan, combine meat and lemon juice; cook over medium heat for 10 minutes, until meat is tender
- Add onions with 3/4 cup of water; continue to cook for another 5 minutes
- Add cauliflower and 5 cups of water; cook over medium heat for 20 minutes until cauliflower is tender; stir occasionally
- Reduce heat, add cilantro; cover and cook over low heat for 5 minutes
- Turn stove off, add flaxseed and stir twice
- Ready to serve

Nutritional Goal

The purpose of modification is to reduce calories, to balance proportion of macronutrients, to improve fat quality, to reduce sodium content, and to enrich food with fiber and nutrients. Calorie content of the healthy recipe is reduced by half, as compared to calorie content of the traditional recipe. In the healthy recipe, calories from macronutrients are balanced by reducing fat and protein along with increasing carbohydrate, as calories from macronutrients charts show. This is achieved by increasing cauliflower and reducing meat in the healthy recipe. The reduction of meat and substitution of corn oil for flaxseed lead to improvement in quality of fat in the healthy recipe. Saturated fat, cholesterol, and trans fatty acid are reduced by more than 80%, when compared to their levels in the traditional recipe. A comparison between nutritional analysis of the traditional and the healthy recipes shows that the healthy recipe has greater nutritional values. Fiber content of the healthy recipe is as twice as the fiber content of the traditional recipe. Thiamin, folate, vitamin C, vitamin A, and magnesium are also increased by more than 100% in the healthy recipe. Calcium and potassium are increased by more than 40% as well. The healthy recipe is highly recommended for individuals with constipation, high lipid profiles, high blood pressure, osteoporosis, post menopause, malnutrition, and excessive body weight.

Nutrient Content	Traditional Recipe	Healthy Recipe
Portion	1 cup	1 cup
Weight (g)	240	264
Kilocalories (kcal)	485	175.5
Protein (g)	22	9.7
Carbohydrate (g)	7	33.4
Fat (g)	41.6	4.3
Saturated Fat (g)	10	0.8
Monounsaturated Fat (g)	13.2	1
Polyunsaturated Fat (g)	15.5	2.3
Trans Fatty Acid (g)	1	0.07
Cholesterol (g)	72.8	12.4
Omega-6 Linoleic (g)	15	0.08
Omega-3 Linolenic (g)	0.3	1.8
Fiber (g)	2.5	6.9
Sugar (g)	2.8	10.6
Water (L)	0.2	0.9
Thiamin (mg)	0.1	0.32
Riboflavin (mg)	0.2	0.18
Niacin (mg)	5.5	2.4
Vitamin B6 (mg)	0.6	0.56
Vitamin B12 (mcg)	2.3	0.45
Folate (DFE) mcg	60.6	121.9
Vitamin C (mg)	38.5	165.3
Vitamin D (mcg)	0	0
Vitamin A (RAE) (mcg)	29.3	78.2
Vitamin E (mg)	4.5	0.7
Calcium (mg)	42	77.9
Iron (mg)	3	2.2
Magnesium (mg)	35.4	72.6
Potassium (mg)	609	871
Zinc (mg)	5.1	2
Sodium (mg)	95.3	53

Portion 1 Cup

Number of Exchanges

Traditional Recipe
1/2 non-starchy vegetable exchange
3 1/3 meat exchange (high fat)
5 2/3 fat exchange (PUFA)

Healthy Recipe
1 non-starchy vegetable exchange
2/3 meat exchange (lean meat)
3 fat exchange (Omega-3-FA)

Calories from Macronutrients

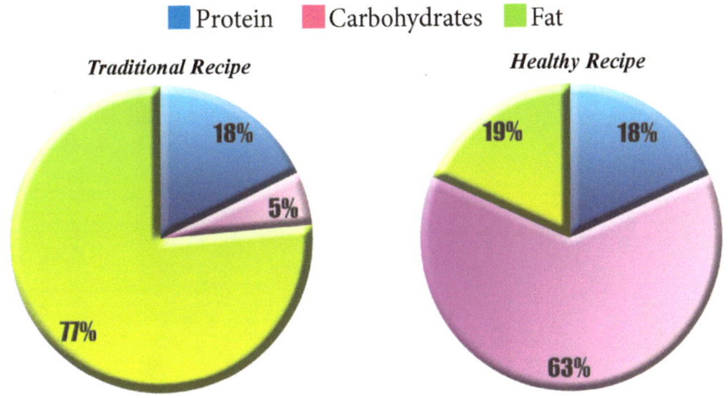

% Fiber Intake Compared to Average Daily Needs

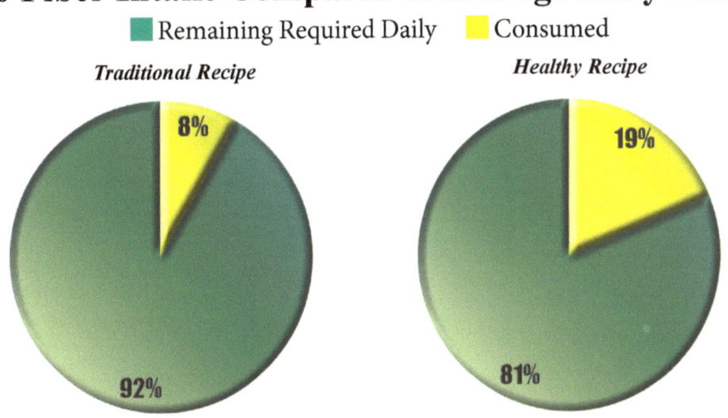

Recommended Portion Sizes & Meal Combinations

Traditional Recipe
(Calorie Controlled)

Men
1 1/4 cups of qarnabit monazal
2 slices of small white pita bread

Women
3/4 cup of qarnabit monazal
1 slice of small white pita bread

Healthy Recipe
(Calorie Controlled & Content Balanced)

Men
3 cups of qarnabit monazal
2 slices of small whole wheat pita bread
1 cup of lowfat ayran

Women
1 3/4 cups of qarnabit monazal
2 slices of small whole wheat pita bread
1 cup of lowfat ayran

Number of Exchanges in a Balanced Meal

Men
2 1/4 non-starchy vegetable exchange
2 meat exchange (lean meat)
9 fat exchange (Omega-3-FA)
2 grain exchange
1 milk exchange

Women
1 1/3 non-starchy vegetable exchange
1 meat exchange (lean meat)
5 1/4 fat exchange (Omega-3-FA)
2 grain exchange
1 milk exchange

Cauliflower Stewed with Meat in Tomato Base

(Toubsi Qarnabit)

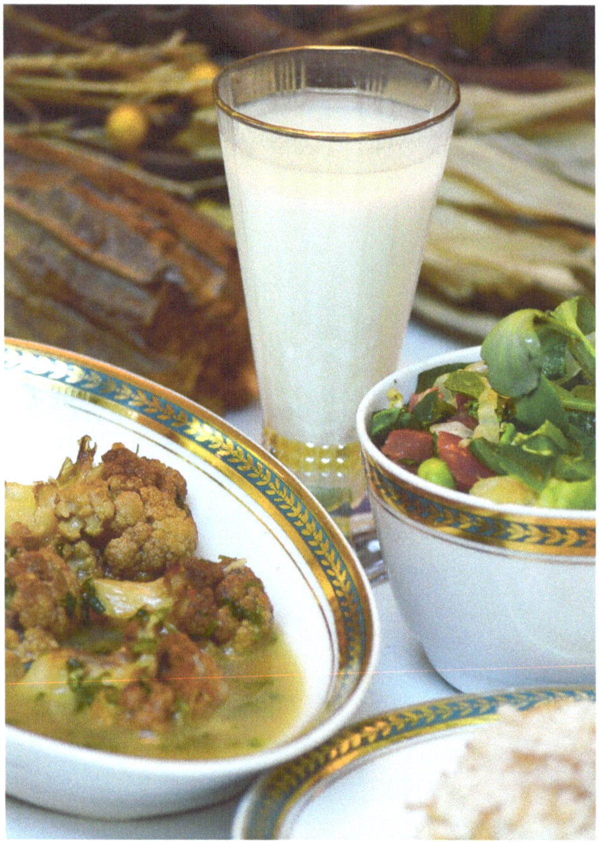

Traditional Recipe, 4 Servings, 4 Cups:

1 cup Chopped Cauliflower~173.6g
5 oz. Ground Meat~143g
1/4 cup Chopped Onions~37.2g
2 Tablespoons Fresh Cilantro~25g
3/4 cup Tomato Paste~216.5g
1/2 teaspoon Black Pepper~1g
4 Tablespoon Corn Oil~56g
3 1/3 cups Meat Broth~679.8g
10 cups Water

Traditional Method of Preparation:

- Season meat with black pepper
- Wash, drain, and chop cauliflower
- In a cooking pan, heat oil and fry onions over medium heat for 5 minutes
- Combine meat with onions; continue cooking for 5 minutes, until meat is tender
- Add cauliflower and continue to cook; stir frequently for 5 minutes
- Add 10 cups of water and tomato paste; stir thoroughly for 2 minutes
- Cook over medium heat for another 30 minutes, until paste forms and cauliflower is tender; stir occasionally
- Reduce heat, add cilantro; cover and cook over low heat for 5 minutes
- Ready to serve

Healthy Recipe, 4 Servings, 4 Cups:

3/4 cup Chopped Cauliflower~159.9g
1 oz. Lean Ground Meat~29g
1/3 cup Chopped Onions~48g
2 3/4 Tablespoons Fresh Cilantro~37g
1 Tablespoon Tomato Paste~18g
1/3 teaspoon Black pepper~0.7g
2 1/4 Tablespoons Ground Flaxseed~16.6g
1 1/3 cups Lemon Juice~342g
2/3 cups Chopped Tomatoes~155.3g
3 1/3 cups Water

Healthy Method of Preparation:

- Season meat with black pepper
- Wash, drain, and chop cauliflower
- In a cooking pan, combine meat and lemon juice; cook over medium heat for 5 minutes until meat is browned
- Add onions with 1/3 cup of water; continue to cook for another 5 minutes
- Combine cauliflower, tomato paste, tomatoes, with 3 cups of water; cover and cook over medium heat for 20 minutes until paste forms and cauliflower is tender; stir occasionally
- Reduce heat, add cilantro, cover and cook over low heat for 5 minutes
- Turn off stove, add flaxseed; stir twice
- Ready to serve

Nutritional Goal

Modification of this recipe aims to reduce calories, to improve quality of fat, to balance proportion of macronutrients, and to enrich food with fiber and nutrients. Calorie content of the healthy recipe is reduced by more than 70%, when compared to calorie content of traditional recipe. Quality of fat is greatly improved in the healthy recipe, when compared to quality of fat in the traditional recipe. Hence, trans fatty acid is totally eliminated; saturated fat and cholesterol are reduced by more than 90%. In the healthy recipe, total fat and protein are reduced, in contrast to carbohydrate that is increased resulting in a more balanced proportion of macronutrients in healthy recipe. The replacement of tomato paste for tomato and tomato juice results in a great reduction in sodium content, more than 90%, in the healthy recipe as compared to sodium content in the traditional recipe. A comparison between nutritional analysis of the traditional and the healthy recipe shows that the healthy recipe contains higher levels of folate and vitamin C. The healthy recipe is recommended to individuals with excessive body weight, high blood pressure, high lipid profiles, and diabetes.

Nutrient Content	Traditional Recipe	Healthy Recipe
Portion	1 cup	1 cup
Weight (g)	256	248
Kilocalories (kcal)	322.9	79.2
Protein (g)	16.28	3.9
Carbohydrate (g)	13.9	14.7
Fat (g)	23.5	2.2
Saturated Fat (g)	5.48	0.3
Monounsaturated Fat (g)	7.45	0.47
Polyunsaturated Fat (g)	8.6	1.3
Trans Fatty Acid (g)	0.5	0
Cholesterol (g)	39.8	2.2
Omega-6 Linoleic (g)	8.43	0.07
Omega-3 Linolenic (g)	0.168	0.98
Fiber (g)	3.86	3.6
Sugar (g)	8	5.3
Water (L)	6	13
Thiamin (mg)	0.09	0.15
Riboflavin (mg)	0.25	0.089
Niacin (mg)	6	1.23
Vitamin B6 (mg)	0.45	0.25
Vitamin B12 (mcg)	1.39	0.18
Folate (DFE) mcg	40.39	52.4
Vitamin C (mg)	34.3	67.2
Vitamin D (mcg)	0	0
Vitamin A (RAE) (mcg)	273	158.4
Vitamin E (mg)	4.4	0.6
Calcium (mg)	55.4	41.6
Iron (mg)	3.5	1
Magnesium (mg)	46.26	38.37
Potassium (mg)	994	489.6
Zinc (mg)	3.14	0.88
Sodium (mg)	1036	59.8

Portion 1 Cup

Number of Exchanges

Traditional Recipe
3/4 non-starchy vegetable exchange
1 meat exchange (high fat)
3 fat exchange (PUFA)

Healthy Recipe
2/3 non-starchy vegetable exchange
1/4 meat exchange (lean meat)
1 2/3 fat exchange (Omega-3-FA)

Calories from Macronutrients

Protein Carbohydrates Fat

Traditional Recipe

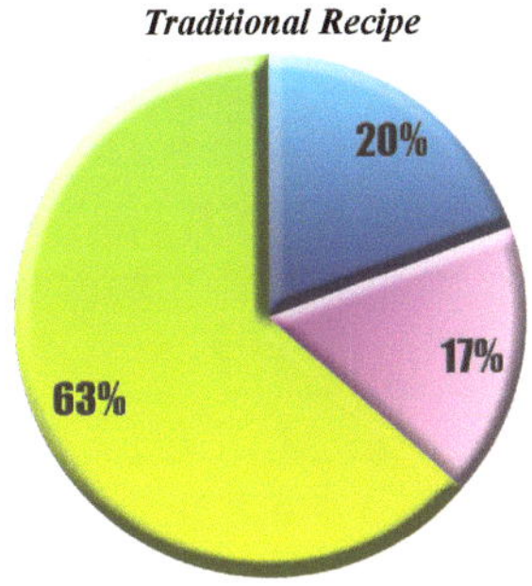

Healthy Recipe

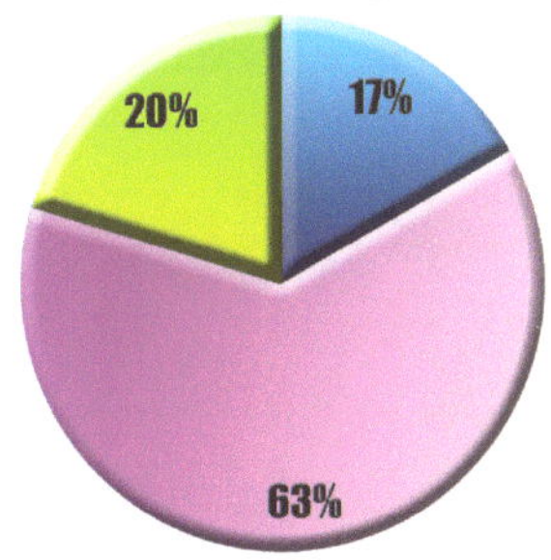

% Fiber Intake Compared to Average Daily Needs

Remaining Required Daily Consumed

Traditional Recipe

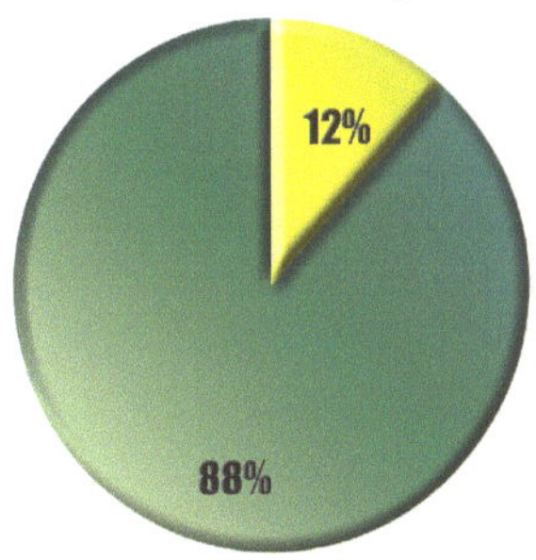

Healthy Recipe

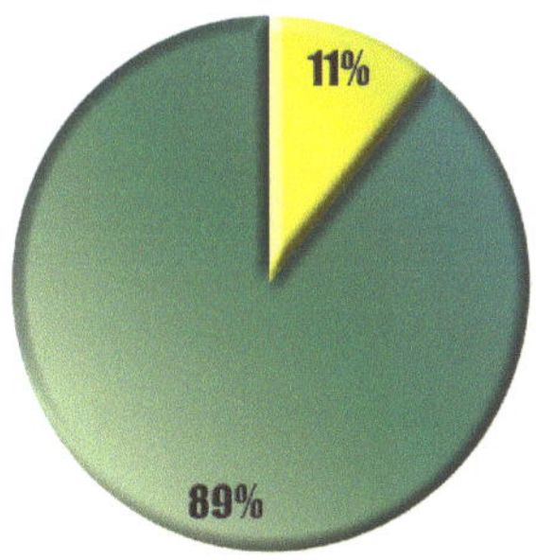

Recommended Portion Sizes & Meal Combinations

Traditional Recipe
(Calorie Controlled)

Men
1 cup of toubsi qarnabit
3/4 cup of traditional egg noodle rice

Women
2/3 cup of toubsi qarnabit
1/2 cup of traditional egg noodle rice

Healthy Recipe
(Calorie Controlled & Content Balanced)

Men
4 cups of toubsi qarnabit
3/4 cup of egg noodle rice (see page:128)
2 cups of green salad-drizzled with vinegar
1 cup of lowfat ayran

Women
2 cups of toubsi qarnabit
1/2 cup of egg noodle rice (see page:128)
1 cup of green salad-drizzled with vinegar
1 cup of lowfat ayran

Number of Exchanges in a Balanced Meal

Men
4 2/3 non-starchy vegetable exchange
1 meat exchange (lean meat)
7 1/3 fat exchange
(1 PUFA, 6 1/3 Omega-3-FA)
3 grain exchange
1 milk exchange

Women
2 1/4 non-starchy vegetable exchange
1/2 meat exchange (lean meat)
4 fat exchange
(3/4 PUFA, 3 1/4 Omega-3-FA)
2 grain exchange
1 milk exchange

Eggplant Stewed with Ground Meat
(Monazal Bazenjan)

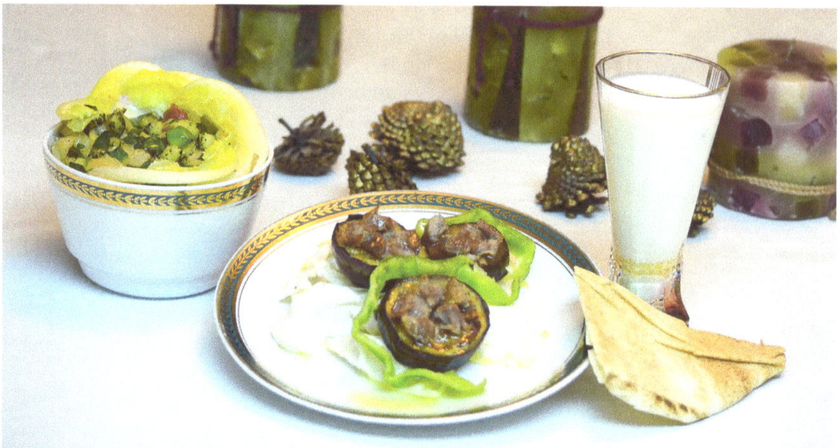

Traditional Recipe, 4 Servings, 4 Cups:

7 oz. Regular Ground Meat~224g
1 cup Chopped Onions~160g
4 cups Eggplant~568g
1 2/3 cups Corn Oil~352g
3 Tablespoons Black Pepper~18g
2 cups Water

Traditional Method of Preparation:

- Cut eggplant into 4 pieces, horizontally
- Heat 2 1/2 tablespoons of oil and fry onions over medium heat for 4 minutes, until onions are golden brown
- Season meat with black pepper, add to onions, and continue to cook over medium heat for another 7 minutes, until meat is brown
- Deep fry eggplant over high heat for 5 minutes, until eggplant is pinkish gold
- Place eggplant in a cooking pan; top every piece with pan-fried meat
- Add 2 cups of water, cover, and cook for 10 minutes until water evaporates
- Ready to serve

Healthy Recipe, 4 Servings, 4 Cups:

5.5 oz. Lean Ground Meat~156g
3/4 cup Chopped Onions~120g
3 cups Eggplant~426g
2 1/4 Tablespoons Corn Oil~30g
4 teaspoons Black Pepper~8g
2 teaspoons Red Chili powder~5.2g
1/3 cup Lemon Juice~74g
1/4 cup Ground Flaxseed~30g
2 cups Water

Healthy Method of Preparation:

- Cut eggplant into 4 pieces horizantally, and place in steamer at high heat for 20 minutes
- Season meat with red chili and black pepper
- In a non-stick skillet, add onions with 2/3 cup of water Bring it to boil and cook over medium heat, until onions are juicy and thick
- Combine lemon juice with onions; stir twice and add meat Continue to cook over medium heat for 7 minutes, until meat is brown
- Add flaxseed and stir twice
- In a cooking pan, place eggplant pieces, brush with oil, top pieces with broiled meat and garnish meat with oil
- Add 2 cups of water, cover and cook over medium heat for 5 minutes
- Ready to serve

Nutritional Goal

The modification of this food is essential since fat is 90% predominant in the traditional recipe. Healthful changes aim to reduce calories, to improve fat quality, and to enrich food with important nutrients. The calorie content of the healthy recipe is reduced by more than 75% when compared to the calorie content of the traditional recipe. The healthy cooking method preserves the quantity and quality of fat; total fat and saturated fat are reduced by more than 80%, when cholesterol and trans fatty acid are reduced by more than 30 % and 60% respectively. The addition of flax seed improves the proportion of omega-6: omega-3 as well supporting the heart health. Nutritional analysis comparison between two recipes shows that the healthy recipe contains more than 10% fiber in addition to higher amounts of thiamin, vitamin C, iron, and magnesium. Although nutritional values are added and quality of fat is improved in the healthy recipe, following the recommended meal combination is necessary to compensate the high fat content and to ensure adequate intake of macronutrients.

Nutrient Content	Traditional Recipe	Healthy Recipe
Portion	1 cup	1 cup
Weight (g)	232	204
Kilocalories (kcal)	933	202.83
Protein (g)	12	11.13
Carbohydrate (g)	11.9	13
Fat (g)	95	12.8
Saturated Fat (g)	14.5	2.15
Monounsaturated Fat (g)	27.5	3.2
Polyunsaturated Fat (g)	47.6	6.75
Trans Fatty Acid (g)	0.5	0.15
Cholesterol (g)	37.6	24.17
Omega-6 Linoleic (g)	0.28	4.5
Omega-3 Linolenic (g)	1	1.79
Fiber (g)	5.3	6.1
Sugar (g)	4.9	4.5
Water (L)	0.2	0.7
Thiamin (mg)	0.1	0.2
Riboflavin (mg)	0.14	0.12
Niacin (mg)	3.5	3.1
Vitamin B6 (mg)	0.4	0.33
Vitamin B12 (mcg)	1.2	0.87
Folate (DFE) mcg	41.3	39.9
Vitamin C (mg)	5.6	14.6
Vitamin D (mcg)	0	0
Vitamin A (RAE) (mcg)	11.6	9.98
Vitamin E (mg)	12.9	1.4
Calcium (mg)	29.5	40.1
Iron (mg)	1.6	1.7
Magnesium (mg)	33	56.85
Potassium (mg)	539	506
Zinc (mg)	2.8	2.5
Sodium (mg)	40.5	31

Portion 1 Cup

Number of Exchanges

Traditional Recipe
1 3/4 meat exchange (medium fat)
1 1/4 non-starchy vegetable exchange
19 1/2 fat exchange (PUFA)

Healthy Recipe
1 1/4 meat exchange (lean)
1 non-starchy vegetable exchange
4 2/3 fat exchange (1 2/3 PUFA, 3 Omega-3-FA)

Calories from Macronutrients

Protein Carbohydrates Fat

Traditional Recipe

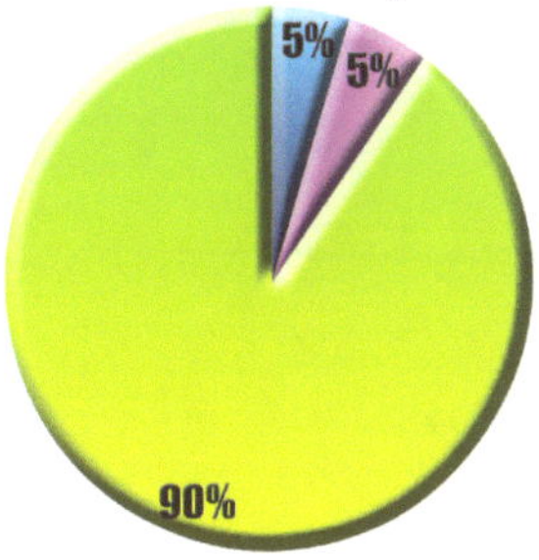

Healthy Recipe

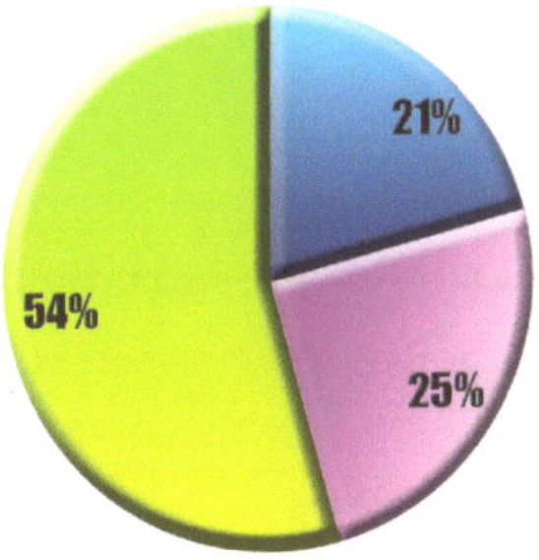

% Fiber Intake Compared to Average Daily Needs

Remaining Required Daily Consumed

Traditional Recipe

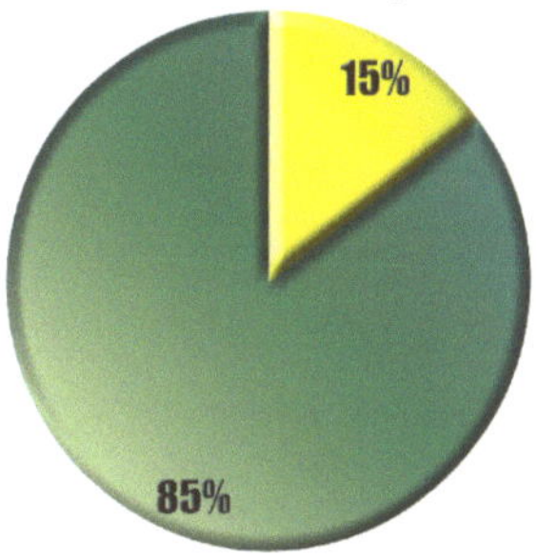

Healthy Recipe

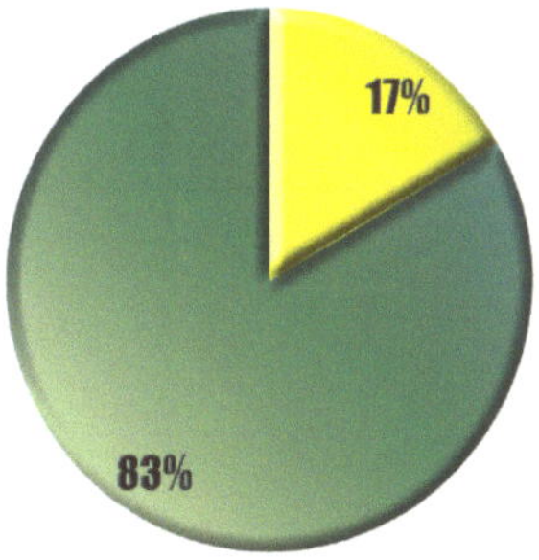

Recommended Portion Sizes & Meal Combinations

Traditional Recipe
(Calorie Controlled)

Men
1/2 cup of monazal eggplant
1/2 cup of traditional egg noodles rice
1/2 cup of regular ayran

Women
1/4 cup of monazal eggplant
1/3 cup of traditional egg noodles rice
1 cup of regular ayran

Healthy Recipe
(Calorie Controlled & Content Balanced)

Men
1 3/4 cups of monazal eggplant
2/3 cup of healthy egg noodles rice (see page:128)
2 cups of green salad-drizzled with vinegar
1 cup of lowfat ayran

Women
1 1/4 cups of monazal eggplant
1/4 cup of healthy egg noodles rice (see page: 128)
1 cup of green salad-drizzled with vinegar

Number of Exchanges in a Balanced Meal

Men
2 meat exchange (lean)
3 3/4 non-starchy vegetable exchange
9 fat exchange (3 3/4 PUFA, 5 1/4 Omega-3-FA)
2 1/2 grain exchange
1 milk exchange

Women
1 2/3 meat exchange (lean)
2 1/4 non-starchy vegetable exchange
6 fat exchange (2 1/3 PUFA, 3 3/4 Omega-3-FA)
1 grain exchange
1 milk exchange

Eggplant Stewed with Meat, Chickpeas & Vegetables

(Mosakaa Bazenjan & Hummus)

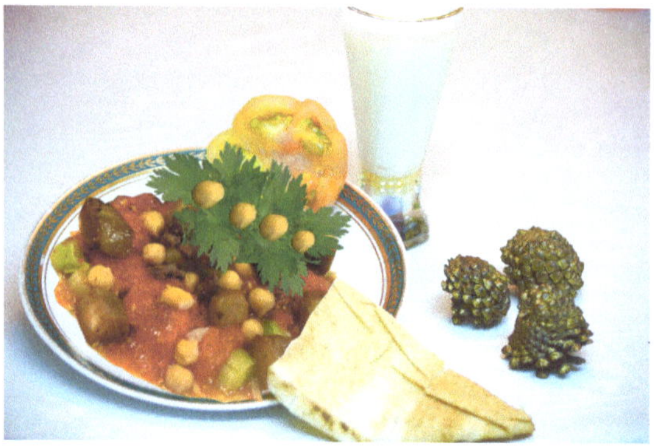

Traditional Recipe, 4 Servings, 4 Cups:

3 cups Peeled Chopped Eggplant~427.6g
1 3/4 Tablespoons Chopped Tomatoes~27g
1/3 cup Soaked Chickpeas~7g
1/3 cup Chopped Onions~64g
2.5 oz. Meat Shank~72.7g
1 1/2 Tablespoons Tomato Paste~24.7g
1 Tablespoon Ground Garlic~4.5g
1/4 cup Chopped Parsley~27.3g
6 3/4 Tablespoons Corn Oil~91g
1/2 teaspoon Black Pepper~1g
4 cups Water

Traditional Method of Preparation:

- Soak chickpeas over night for 12 hours
- Heat oil in a large frying pan, and fry eggplant over high heat for 5 minutes. Turn eggplant carefully with blunt ended tongs to brown evenly
- In a cooking pan, heat 1 tablespoon of oil and fry onions and garlic over medium heat for 5 minutes, until gold
- Season meat with black pepper and combine with onions and garlic; continue cooking for another 5 minutes; stir frequently to prevent sticking
- Add tomatoes and tomato paste; stir twice
- Combine all ingredients together with 4 cups of water, cover and cook over medium heat for 30 minutes, until meat and chickpeas are tender
- Ready to serve

Healthy Recipe, 4 Servings, 4 Cups:

2 1/2 cups Peeled Chopped Eggplant~350.23g
1 1/2 cups Chopped Tomatoes~381g
1 cup Soaked Chickpeas~177g
1/3 cup Chopped Onions~48.5g
0.3 oz. Lean Meat Shank~10.5g
2 Tablespoons Tomato Juice~45g
1 Tablespoon Ground Garlic~14g
2/3 cup Chopped Parsley~62.4g
2 3/4 teaspoons Ground Flaxseed~7g
5 cups Water

Healthy Method of Preparation:

- Soak chickpeas over night for 12 hours
- Steam eggplant at high heat for 20 minutes
- In a cooking pan, bring 5 cups of water to boil
- Season meat with black pepper and cook over medium heat for 5 minutes
- Add chickpeas with meat and continue cooking for another 15 minutes, until chickpeas are tender
- Combine steamed eggplant, onions, tomatoes, tomato juice, garlic, and parsley with meat and chickpeas
- Cook over medium heat for 10 minutes
- Turn stove off; add flaxseed and stir twice
- Ready to serve

Nutritional Goal

The purpose of the modification is to reduce calories, to balance proportion of macronutrients, to improve quality of fat and omega-6: omega-3 ratio, to reduce sodium content, and to enrich food with fiber and nutrients. It is essential to modify this recipe since calories from fat are predominant in the traditional recipe. The calorie content of the healthy recipe is reduced by more than 25%, when compared to the calorie content of the traditional recipe. In the healthy recipe, fat is reduced by more than 75%, as protein and carbohydrate are increased by more than 30% and 80% respectively in order to balance the proportion of macronutrients. Saturated fat and cholesterol are reduced by more than 75% in the healthy recipe, when compared to their levels in the traditional recipe. The addition of flaxseed and parsley improves the proportion of omega-6: omega-3 in the healthy recipe. A comparison between nutrient contents of the traditional and the healthy recipes shows that the healthy recipe contains higher levels of different nutrients. Fiber, folate, iron, magnesium, zinc, and potassium are enriched by more than half in the healthy recipe. In contrast, the level of sodium content is reduced by more than 10%. The healthy recipe is recommended to individuals with constipation, high lipid profiles, high blood pressure, malnutrition, and excessive body weight.

Nutrient Content	Traditional Recipe	Healthy Recipe
Portion	1 cup	1 cup
Weight (g)	232	228
Kilocalories (kcal)	326.6	229
Protein (g)	8.3	11.9
Carbohydrate (g)	20.7	40
Fat (g)	24.7	4
Saturated Fat (g)	3.3	0.5
Monounsaturated Fat (g)	6.8	0.9
Polyunsaturated Fat (g)	13	1.5
Trans Fatty Acid (g)	0	0
Cholesterol (g)	5.6	0.8
Omega-6 Linoleic (g)	0.1	0.2
Omega-3 Linolenic (g)	0.3	0.5
Fiber (g)	7.5	13.1
Sugar (g)	6.1	10
Water (L)	12.6	17.5
Thiamin (mg)	0.2	0.34
Riboflavin (mg)	0.1	0.18
Niacin (mg)	2	2.3
Vitamin B6 (mg)	0.3	0.5
Vitamin B12 (mcg)	0.5	0.08
Folate (DFE) mcg	138.6	309.9
Vitamin C (mg)	16	40.5
Vitamin D (mcg)	0	0
Vitamin A (RAE) (mcg)	229	649.6
Vitamin E (mg)	3.8	1
Calcium (mg)	49	100.4
Iron (mg)	2.4	4.5
Magnesium (mg)	46	91.8
Potassium (mg)	600	979.6
Zinc (mg)	2	2.3
Sodium (mg)	69	58.9

Portion 1 Cup

Number of Exchanges

Traditional Recipe
1 non-starchy vegetable exchange
2/3 meat exchange (2/3 high fat)
5 fat exchange (PUFA)

Healthy Recipe
1 1/4 non-starchy vegetable exchange
1/2 meat exchange (1/2 very lean)
3/4 fat exchange (Omega-3-FA)
1/2 starch exchange

Calories from Macronutrients

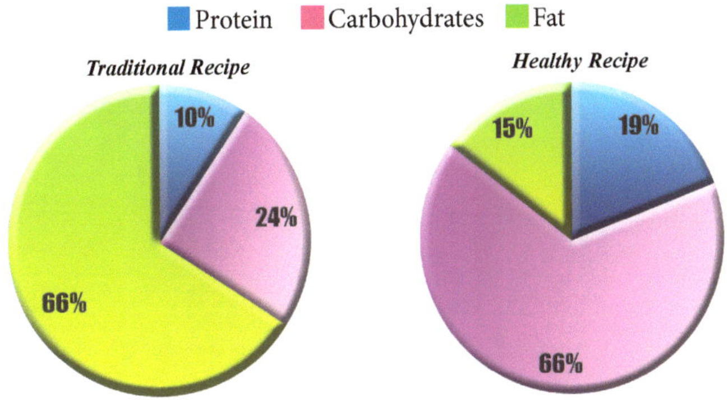

% Fiber Intake Compared to Average Daily Needs

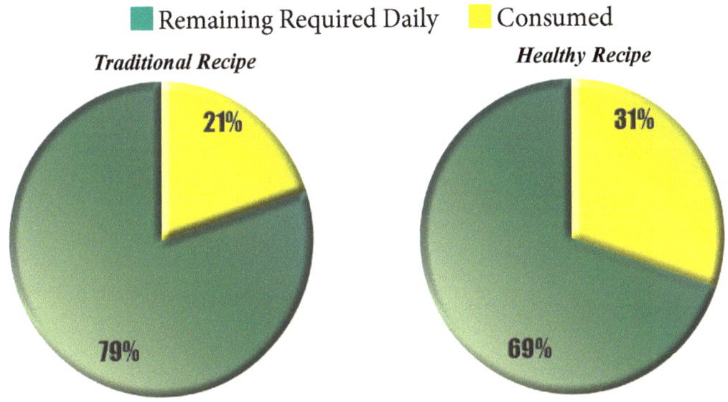

Recommended Portion Sizes & Meal Combinations

Traditional Recipe
(Calorie Controlled)

Men
2 cups of mosakaa bazenjan and hummus
1 1/2 slice of small white pita bread

Women
1 1/4 cups of mosakaa bazenjan and hummus
1 slice of small white pita bread

Healthy Recipe
(Calorie Controlled & Content Balanced)

Men
2 1/4 cups of mosakaa bazenjan and hummus
2 slice of small whole wheat pita bread
1 cup of lowfat ayran

Women
1 1/2 cups of mosakaa bazenjan and hummus
1 slice of small whole wheat pita bread
1 cup of lowfat ayran

Number of Exchanges in a Balanced Meal

Men
3 non-starchy vegetable exchange
1 meat exchange (very lean)
1 1/2 fat exchange (Omega-3-FA)
1 starch exchange
2 grain exchange
1 milk exchange

Women
2 non-starchy vegetable exchange
3/4 meat exchange (very lean)
1 fat exchange (Omega-3-FA)
3/4 starch exchange
1 grain exchange
1 milk exchange

Meatless Eggplant Stewed with Tomatoes

(Mosakaa)

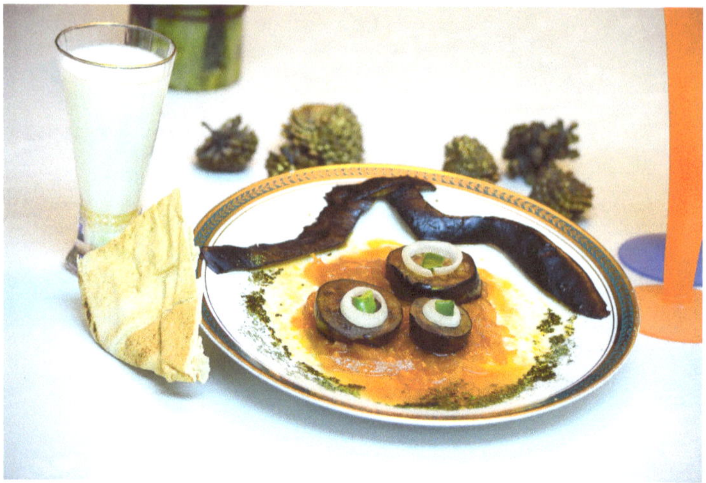

Traditional Recipe, 4 Servings, 4 Cups:

4 3/4 cups Thick Eggplant Slices~463.52g
3 cups Thick Tomato Slices~752g
2 Tablespoons Ground Garlic~24g
5 1/2 cups Shredded Onions~888g
1 3/4 cups Corn Oil~399.84g
*Optional: 1 1/3 cups chopped green pepper~176g

Traditional Method of Preparation:

- Heat oil in a large frying pan, add sliced eggplants and fry over high heat for 5 minutes; turn eggplant carefully with blunt ended tongs to brown evenly
- Pre-heat oven at high heat for 10 minutes
- In oven dish, place tomato slices and shredded onions on the base; layer and arrange fried eggplant; sprinkle garlic on the top
- Place dish in oven at medium heat for 15 minutes and remove
- Ready to serve

Healthy Recipe, 4 Servings, 4 Cups:

4 cups Thick Eggplant Slices~386.744g
1 1/2 cups Thick Tomato Slices~370.074g
1/2 teaspoon Ground Garlic~2g
1/2 cup Shredded Onions~86.68g
3 1/3 teaspoons Corn Oil~15g
1 2/3 cups Water
*Optional: 2 cups fresh green pepper freshly cut aside

Healthy Method of Preparation:

- Steam eggplant and tomatoes for 20 minutes
- In a medium pan, add shredded onions to 1/2 cup of cold water
- Bring it to a boil and cook for 10 minutes until onions are thick and juicy
- In oven dish, place cooked onions on the base and arrange steamed tomatoes and eggplants over onions; sprinkle garlic on the top
- Add 1 1/4 cups of water; place in oven at high heat and cook for 30 minutes
- Turn oven off; drizzle corn oil over eggplants
- Ready to serve

Nutritional Goal

The modification of this recipe is important because the traditional recipe has surplus high calories with multiple negative health impacts. A cup of the traditional recipe meets approximately 75% of women daily needs and 50% of men daily needs. The negative health impacts are due to the cooking method, (frying and oil heating). Frying food converts the good fat into bad fat. Although the proportion of macronutrients is not well-balanced in the healthy recipe; it is much healthier, when compared to the proportion of macronutrients of the traditional recipe. The calorie content of the healthy recipe is reduced by more than 80%, when compared to calorie content of the traditional recipe. Also, great reduction in total fat and saturated fat is obtained; they are reduced by more than 80%, and trans fatty acid is roughly eliminated in the healthy recipe. The nutritional analysis shows that the traditional recipe is richer in a variety of nutrients; however, it is not nutritionally balanced. Following the suggested meal combination is necessary in order to balance the entire meal and obtain most of the health benefits. The healthy recipe is recommended to individuals with excessive body weight and constipation.

Nutrient Content	Traditional Recipe	Healthy Recipe
Portion	1 cup	1 cup
Weight (g)	166	219
Kilocalories (kcal)	1056.3	82.3
Protein (g)	5.6	2
Carbohydrate (g)	40.4	11.5
Fat (g)	100.8	4
Saturated Fat (g)	12.9	0.6
Monounsaturated Fat (g)	24.4	1
Polyunsaturated Fat (g)	59.2	2.4
Trans Fatty Acid (g)	0.3	0.01
Cholesterol (g)	0	0
Omega-6 Linoleic (g)	58.3	2.35
Omega-3 Linolenic (g)	0.7	0.04
Fiber (g)	10.2	4.7
Sugar (g)	18	5.6
Water (L)	0.53	0.2
Thiamin (mg)	0.3	0.1
Riboflavin (mg)	0.2	0.1
Niacin (mg)	2.3	1.2
Vitamin B6 (mg)	0.7	0.2
Vitamin B12 (mcg)	0	0
Folate (DFE) mcg	100.9	39
Vitamin C (mg)	77.9	15
Vitamin D (mcg)	0	0
Vitamin A (RAE) (mcg)	535	241.5
Vitamin E (mg)	18.3	1
Calcium (mg)	93	24
Iron (mg)	1.5	0.5
Magnesium (mg)	65	26
Potassium (mg)	1132.8	475
Zinc (mg)	1	0.35
Sodium (mg)	21	7.3

Portion 1 Cup

Number of Exchanges

Traditional Recipe
3 2/3 non-starchy vegetable exchange
22 1/4 fat exchange (PUFA)

Healthy Recipe
1 1/2 non-starchy vegetable exchange
1 fat exchange (PUFA)

Calories from Macronutrients

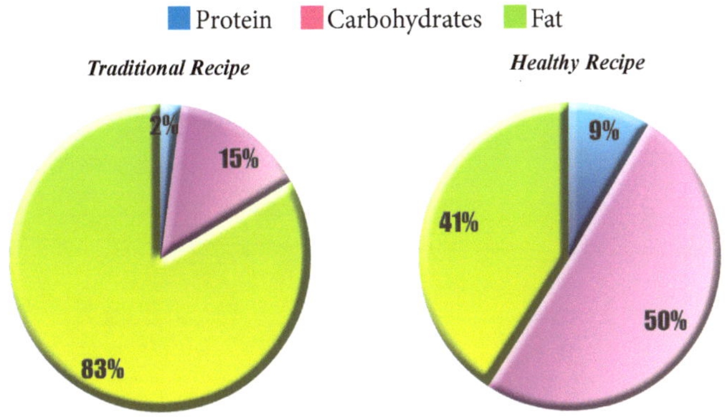

% Fiber Intake Compared to Average Daily Needs

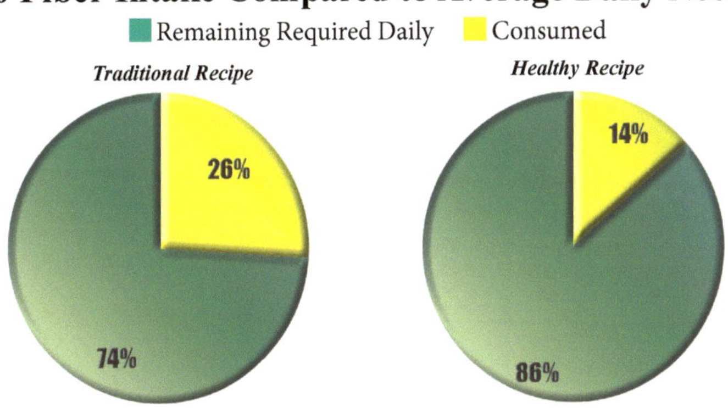

Recommended Portion Sizes & Meal Combinations

Traditional Recipe
(Calorie Controlled)

Men
2/3 cup of mosakaa
1 1/4 slices of small white pita bread

Women
6 1/2 Tablespoons of mosakaa
1 slice of small white pita bread

Healthy Recipe
(Calorie Controlled & Content Balanced)

Men
4 1/2 cups of mosakaa
4 slices of small whole wheat pita bread
1 cup of lowfat ayran

Women
3 cups of mosakaa
2 slices of small whole wheat pita bread
1 cup of lowfat ayran

Number of Exchanges in a Balanced Meal

Men
6 3/4 non-starchy vegetable exchange
3 2/3 fat exchange (PUFA)
4 grain exchange
1 milk exchange

Women
4 1/2 non-starchy vegetable exchange
2 1/3 fat exchange (PUFA)
2 grain exchange
1 milk exchange

Fava Bean Stewed with Ground Meat

(Mofarakah Be Al Foul)

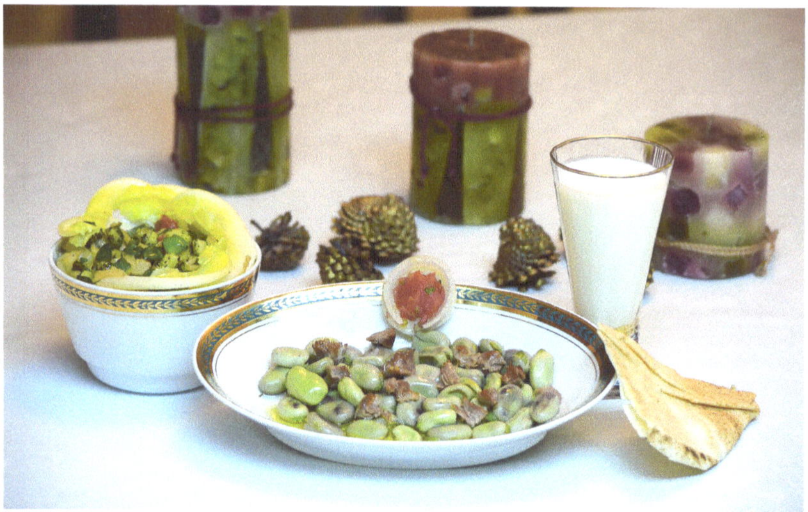

Traditional Recipe, 4 Servings, 4 Cups:

1 2/3 cups Fresh Fava Beans~319.5g
7 oz. Ground Meat~202.35g
6 Tablespoons Chopped Onions~60.35g
4 1/2 Tablespoons Corn Oil~64.36g
2 cups Water

Traditional Method of Preparation:

- Sprinkle meat with black pepper
- Wash and drain fava bean
- Heat oil and fry onions over medium heat for 5 minutes
- Combine meat with onions; continue cooking for 8-10 minutes, until meat is brown
- Add beans to meat and onions; stir thoroughly for 2 minutes
- Add 2 cups of water; cover and cook over medium heat for 20 minutes; stir occasionally to prevent sticking
- Ready to serve

Healthy Recipe, 4 Servings, 4 Cups:

2 1/3 cups Fresh Fava Beans~466.78g
2.75 oz. Lean Meat~76.75g
1 2/3 cups Chopped Onions~257.25g
3 Tablespoons Corn Oil~43.2g
4 cups Water

Healthy Method of Preparation:

- Sprinkle meat with black pepper
- In a cooking pan, simmer meat with 3 cups of water over high heat for 10 minutes
- Add fava beans to meat, stir twice for 5 minutes
- In a saucepan, bring onions with 1 cup of water to a boil over medium heat for 10 minutes
- Add olive oil and reduce to a low heat; stir frequently for 30 seconds
- Combine sautéed onions with meat and beans; stir frequently for 1 minute over low heat
- Ready to serve

Nutritional Goal

Although both recipes have same caloric contents, calories from macronutrients are more balanced in the healthy recipe. The modification aims to improve fat content, and to enrich food with fiber and nutrients. Total fat and trans fatty acid are reduced by more than 30% and 45% in the healthy recipe, when compared to their levels in the traditional recipe. The change in meat:onion and beans ratio leads to significant enrichments of fiber in the healthy recipe. A comparison between the nutritional analysis of the recipes shows that fiber is increased by half in the healthy recipe. Calcium, magnesium, zinc, iron, vitamin C and potassium are increased by more than 40% in the healthy recipe. Folate is also increased by more than 75%, when other B vitamins are increased by more than half. In addition, the healthy recipe contains five times less sodium than the traditional recipe. The healthy recipe is recommended to athletes and individuals with osteoporosis, malnutrition, hypertension, and nerve disorders.

Nutrient Content	Traditional Recipe	Healthy Recipe
Portion	1 cup	1 cup
Weight (g)	132.4	224
Kilocalories (kcal)	303.62	298.4
Protein (g)	14.3	21.6
Carbohydrate (g)	11.08	19.88
Fat (g)	22.7	14.8
Saturated Fat (g)	4.6	3.06
Monounsaturated Fat (g)	6.6	4.07
Polyunsaturated Fat (g)	9.8	6.8
Trans Fatty Acid (g)	0.44	0.26
Cholesterol (g)	33.4	42.19
Omega-6 Linoleic (g)	9.5	6.33
Omega-3 Linolenic (g)	0.28	0.34
Fiber (g)	3.6	5.7
Sugar (g)	2.06	4.78
Water (L)	0.11	50.19
Thiamin (mg)	0.167	0.26
Riboflavin (mg)	0.17	0.257
Niacin (mg)	3.64	5.5
Vitamin B6 (mg)	0.23	1.53
Vitamin B12 (mcg)	1.09	1.53
Folate (DFE) mcg	5.9	15.46
Vitamin C (mg)	27.2	42.04
Vitamin D (mcg)	0	0
Vitamin A (RAE) (mcg)	84.35	122.45
Vitamin E (mg)	2.7	2.15
Calcium (mg)	29.9	45.42
Iron (mg)	2.8	3.93
Magnesium (mg)	42	65.1
Potassium (mg)	380	615.27
Zinc (mg)	2.8	4.24
Sodium (mg)	584.97	104.5

Portion 1 Cup

Number of Exchanges

Traditional Recipe
1 starch exchange
2 3/4 meat exchange
(1 very lean, 1 2/3 medium fat)
3 1/2 fat exchange (PUFA)

Healthy Recipe
1 starch exchange
3 1/3 meat exchange (1 very lean, 2/3 lean)
2 1/3 fat exchange (PUFA)
1/3 non-starchy vegetable exchange

Calories from Macronutrients

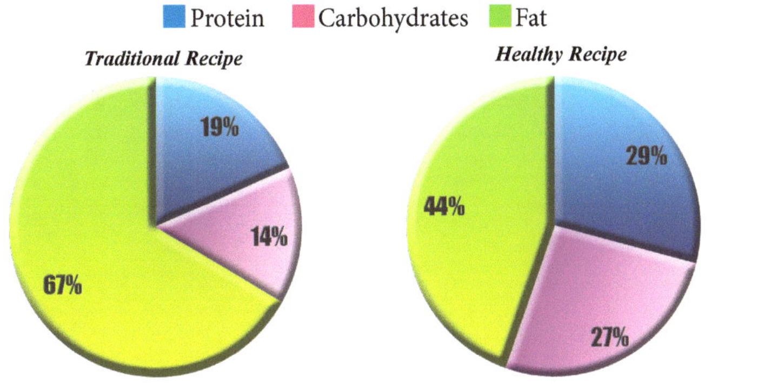

% Fiber Intake Compared to Average Daily Needs

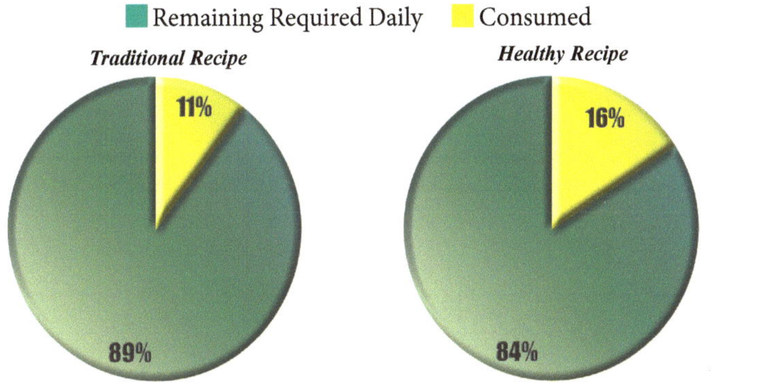

Recommended Portion Sizes & Meal Combinations

Traditional Recipe
(Calorie Controlled)

Men
1 3/4 cups of mofarakah be al foul
1 3/4 slices of small white pita bread
1cup of regular plain yogurt

Women
1 cup of mofarakah be al foul
1 slice of small white pita bread
2/3 cup of regular plain yogurt

Healthy Recipe
(Calorie Controlled & Content Balanced)

Men
1 3/4 cups of mofarakah be al foul
1 slice of small whole wheat pita bread
2 cups of green salad–drizzled with vinegar
1/2 cup of lowfat plain yogurt

Women
1 cup of mofarakah be al foul
1/2 slice of small whole wheat pita bread
1 cup of green salad-drizzled with vinegar
1/2 cup of lowfat plain yogurt

Number of Exchanges in a Balanced Meal

Men
2 starch exchange
3 meat exchange (2 very lean, 1 lean)
2 3/4 non-starchy vegetable exchange
4 1/4 fat exchange (PUFA)
2/3 milk exchange
1 grain exchange

Women
1 starch exchange
1 2/3 meat exchange (1 very lean, 2/3 lean)
1 1/3 non-starchy vegetable exchange
2 1/3 fat exchange (PUFA)
2/3 milk exchange
1 grain exchange

Fava Beans Sautéed with Olive Oil & Cilantro

(Appetizer: Foul Moa'ala)

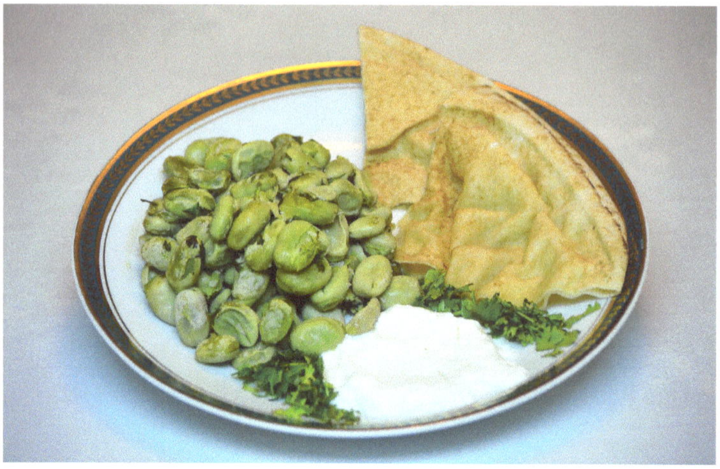

Traditional Recipe, 4 Servings, 4 Cups:

2 2/3 cups Fresh Fava Beans~525g
5 Tablespoons Chopped Cilantro~66g
3 1/4 Tablespoons Ground Garlic~39g
5 3/4 Tablespoons Olive Oil~78g
3 cups Water

Traditional Method of Preparation:

- Bring 3 cups of water to boil and add fava beans for 5 minutes, until fava beans are tender
- Remove fava beans from water and drain
- In a cooking pan, heat olive oil and fry beans and garlic over medium heat for 4 minutes; stir frequently to prevent sticking
- Add cilantro to pan and continue stirring for another 3 minutes
- Ready to serve

Healthy Recipe, 4 Servings, 4 Cups:

3 cups Fresh Fava Beans~588g
6 Tablespoons Chopped Cilantro~78g
5 2/3 Tablespoons Ground Garlic~67.2g
1 Tablespoon Olive Oil~13.2g
1/2 cup Water

Healthy Method of Preparation:

- Steam fava beans at high heat for 20 minutes, until beans are tender
- Add chopped cilantro to beans and continue steaming for 5 minutes
- Transfer beans and cilantro to a cooking pan with 1/2 cup of water and garlic. Cook over medium heat for 5 minutes, until water evaporates
- Place food in serving plate, drizzle with fresh olive oil
- Ready to serve

Nutritional Goal

The purpose of modification is to reduce calories and preserves nutritional values of beans. Calories of the healthy recipe are reduced by more than 25% when compared to calories of the traditional recipe. Also, the healthy recipe is richer in many nutrients than the traditional recipe, due to the change in cooking method. Steaming beans instead of boiling preserves most nutrients such as zinc, potassium, magnesium, calcium, folate, vitamin A, vitamin C, and B complex vitamins. This cooking method also keeps the volume of food; thus, a less amount of beans with much more fiber content is presented in the healthy recipe. Adding the oil at the end of the cooking preserves the nutritional quality of oil and avoids the transition of fat into trans fatty acid by heating the oil. The analysis of calories from macronutrients shows that the healthy recipe is well-balanced and highly recommended to individuals with diabetes, excessive body weight, high lipid profiles, osteoporosis, and malnutrition.

Nutrient Content	Traditional Recipe	Healthy Recipe
Portion	1 cup	1 cup
Weight (g)	190.89	160.5
Kilocalories (kcal)	233.98	168.6
Protein (g)	8.4	9.9
Carbohydrate (g)	19.4	24.4
Fat (g)	14.5	4.4
Saturated Fat (g)	2	0.68
Monounsaturated Fat (g)	10	2.5
Polyunsaturated Fat (g)	1.8	0.86
Trans Fatty Acid (g)	0	0
Cholesterol (g)	0	0
Omega-6 Linoleic (g)	1.45	0.5
Omega-3 Linolenic (g)	0.36	0.3
Fiber (g)	6.1	6.9
Sugar (g)	2.8	3.2
Water (L)	0.12	0.15
Thiamin (mg)	0.28	0.3
Riboflavin (mg)	0.183	0.2
Niacin (mg)	2.22	2.5
Vitamin B6 (mg)	0.186	0.3
Vitamin B12 (mcg)	0	0
Folate (DFE) mcg	8.96	10.7
Vitamin C (mg)	47.75	55.6
Vitamin D (mcg)	0	0
Vitamin A (RAE) (mcg)	178.75	200
Vitamin E (mg)	1.6	0.65
Calcium (mg)	51.1	72.32
Iron (mg)	3.13	3.56
Magnesium (mg)	55.2	63.44
Potassium (mg)	404.7	484.9
Zinc (mg)	0.96	1.17
Sodium (mg)	68.7	77.3

Portion 1 Cup

Number of Exchanges

Traditional Recipe
1 1/3 starch exchange
1 1/3 meat exchange (very lean)
4 1/3 fat exchange (MUFA)

Healthy Recipe
1 1/2 starch exchange
1 1/2 meat exchange (very lean)
3/4 fat exchange (MUFA)

Calories from Macronutrients

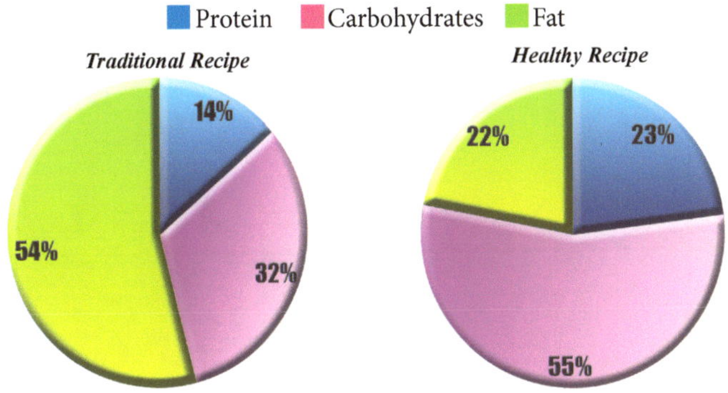

% Fiber Intake Compared to Average Daily Needs

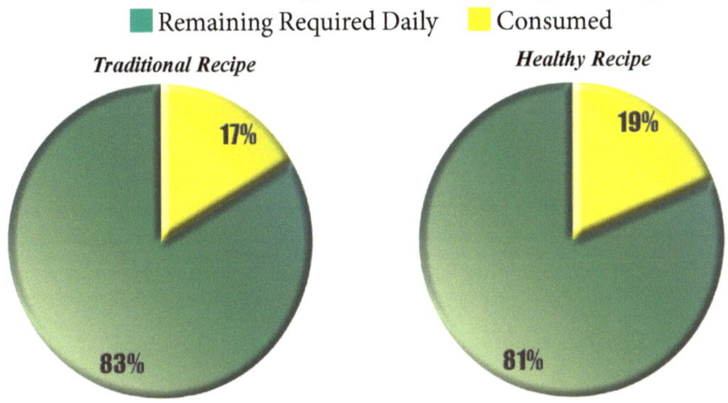

Recommended Portion Sizes & Meal Combinations

Traditional Recipe
(Calorie Controlled)

Men
3/4 cup fava bean sautéed with olive oil & cilantro
1 small white pita bread
1/2 cup of regular plain yogurt

Women
1/3 cup fava bean sautéed with olive oil & cilantro
1/2 small white pita bread
1/4 cup of regular plain yogurt

Healthy Recipe
(Calorie Controlled & Content Balanced)

Men
1 cup of fava bean sautéed with olive oil & cilantro
1 small whole wheat pita bread
1/2 cup of lowfat plain yogurt

Women
1/2 cup fava bean sautéed with olive oil & cilantro
1/2 small whole wheat pita bread
1/4 cup of lowfat plain yogurt

Number of Exchanges in a Balanced Meal

Men
1 1/2 starch exchange
1 1/2 meat exchange (very lean)
3/4 fat exchange (MUFA)
1 grain exchange
2/3 milk exchange

Women
3/4 starch exchange
3/4 meat exchange (very lean)
1/3 fat exchange (MUFA)
1/2 grain exchange
1/3 milk exchange

French Green Beans Stewed with Meat in Tomatoe Base & Broth

(Loubyah Matmour)

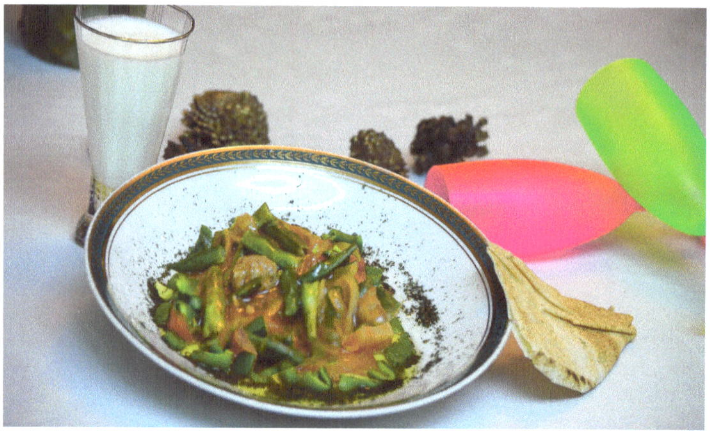

Traditional Recipe, 4 Servings, 4 Cups:

1/3 cup French Cut Green Beans~100.5g
4.8 oz. Shank Meat~136g
1/3 cup Chopped Tomatoes~75.4g
3/4 Tablespoon Chopped Onions~12.5g
3/4 Tablespoon Lemon Juice~13g
1/2 teaspoon Black Pepper~1g
3 1/3 Tablespoons Ghee~43.2g
10 cups Water

Traditional Method of Preparation:

- Heat ghee and fry chopped onions and French cut green beans over medium heat for 5 minutes
- Season meat with black pepper and combine meat with onions and beans
- Continue to fry for another 5 minutes until meat is lightly browned
- Stir constantly to prevent sticking
- Combine all ingredients together with meat broth water
- Cover and cook over medium heat for 30 minutes
- Stir occasionally
- Ready to serve

Healthy Recipe, 4 Servings, 4 Cups:

3/4 cup Steamed French Cut Green Beans~140g
1.4 oz. Lean Shank Meat~41.8g
3/4 cup Chopped Tomatoes~175g
1/3 cup Chopped Onions~70g
1/3 cup Lemon Juice~106.7g
1/2 teaspoon Black Pepper~1g
1 1/3 teaspoons Ground Flaxseed~3.5g
2 cups Tomato Juice~530.8g
6 cups Water

Healthy Method of Preparation:

- Steam French cut green beans at high heat for 15 minutes
- Bring 6 cups of water to boil
- Combine meat and onions over medium heat for 15 minutes
- Add lemon juice, tomato juice, steamed French cut green beans and tomatoes
- Cook over medium heat for another 15 minutes
- Turn stove off, sprinkle ground flaxseed over dish
- Ready to serve

Nutritional Goal

The purpose of modification is to reduce calories to balance the proportion of macronutrients, to improve quality of fat, and to enrich food with fiber and nutrients. Calorie content of the healthy recipe is reduced by more than half when compared to calorie content of the traditional recipe. By reducing meat, omitting ghee, and by increasing tomatoes and French cut green beans, results in the healthier proportion of macronutrients, as calories from the macronutrients charts show. Total fat, saturated fat, and cholesterol are reduced by more than 85% in the healthy recipe when compared to their levels in the traditional recipe. Apparently, the enrichment of the recipe with vegetables adds numerous nutritional values to the healthy recipe when compared to nutritional values of the traditional recipe. Fiber content is increased by more than 200%; vitamin C and zinc are increased by more than 1000%. There is more than 30% increase in levels of B-complex vitamins and iron. Also, potassium, vitamin E, and magnesium are increased by more than 100%. Calcium content of the healthy recipe is increased by more than half. Also, water content is greatly improved by more than 1000%. It does not promote thirst and is recommended to consume during fasting month, Ramadan. It is also recommended to individuals with diabetes, high lipid profiles, osteoporosis, malnutrition, and excessive body weight.

Nutrient Content	Traditional Recipe	Healthy Recipe
Portion	1 cup	1 cup
Weight (g)	223.5	240
Kilocalories (kcal)	425	96.6
Protein (g)	4	6.6
Carbohydrate (g)	2.5	19
Fat (g)	45	1.4
Saturated Fat (g)	28	0.5
Monounsaturated Fat (g)	13	0.5
Polyunsaturated Fat (g)	1.7	0.4
Trans Fatty Acid (g)	0	0
Cholesterol (g)	114.7	2.6
Omega-6 Linoleic (g)	0.03	0.06
Omega-3 Linolenic (g)	0.001	0.2
Fiber (g)	0.7	2.3
Sugar (g)	1.1	6.3
Water (L)	0.4	5.5
Thiamin (mg)	0.02	0.1
Riboflavin (mg)	0.07	0.1
Niacin (mg)	2.5	3.3
Vitamin B6 (mg)	0.05	0.2
Vitamin B12 (mcg)	0.2	0.4
Folate (DFE) mcg	3.8	31.9
Vitamin C (mg)	4.1	80
Vitamin D (mcg)	0	0
Vitamin A (RAE) (mcg)	47.9	119.7
Vitamin E (mg)	1.3	0.3
Calcium (mg)	24	42.8
Iron (mg)	0.7	1
Magnesium (mg)	9.5	27.3
Potassium (mg)	224.6	530.3
Zinc (mg)	0.04	0.7
Sodium (mg)	1009	1016

Portion 1 Cup

Number of Exchanges

Traditional Recipe
1 meat exchange (high fat)
2 1/2 fat exchange (saturated)

Healthy Recipe
1/3 meat exchange (medium fat)
1/3 fat exchange (Omega-3-FA)
1 non-starchy vegetable exchange

Calories from Macronutrients

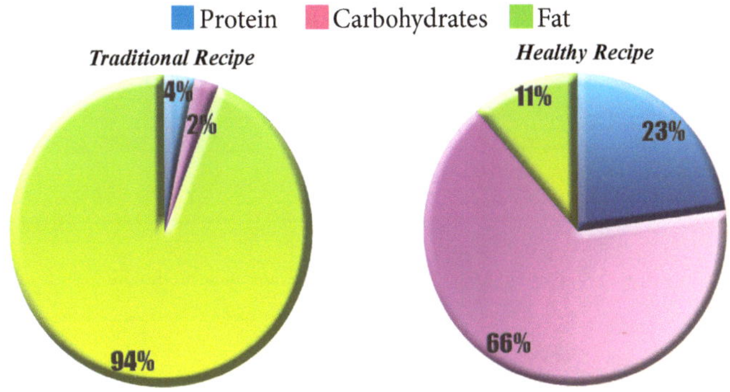

% Fiber Intake Compared to Average Daily Needs

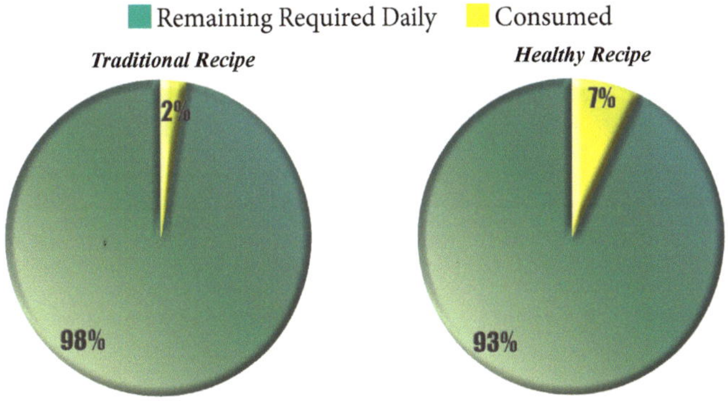

Recommended Portion Sizes & Meal Combinations

Traditional Recipe
(Calorie Controlled)

Men
1 1/2 cups of loubyah matmour
2 slices of small white pita bread

Women
1 cup of loubyah matmour
1 slice of small white pita bread

Healthy Recipe
(Calorie Controlled & Content Balanced)

Men
4 1/2 cups of loubyah matmour
3 slices of small whole pita wheat bread
1 cup of lowfat ayran

Women
2 1/2 cups of loubyah matmour
2 slices of small whole pita wheat bread
1 cup of lowfat ayran

Number of Exchanges in a Balanced Meal

Men
5 non-starchy vegetable exchange
1 1/3 meat exchange (medium fat)
1 1/3 fat exchange (Omega-3-FA)
3 grain exchange
1 milk exchange

Women
3 non-starchy vegetable exchange
3/4 meat exchange (medium fat)
3/4 fat exchange (Omega-3-FA)
2 grain exchange
1 milk exchange

French Green Beans Stewed with Meat in Tomato Base

(Loubyah Maraq)

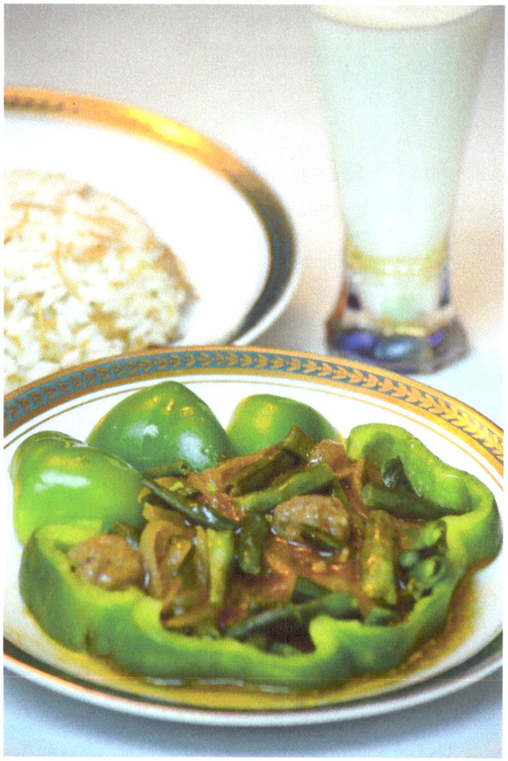

Traditional Recipe, 4 Servings, 4 Cups:

3/4 cup French Cut Green Beans~215g
10.2 oz. Shank Meat~291g
2/3 Chopped Tomatoes~161g
2 3/4 Tablespoons Chopped Onions~27g
1 3/4 Tablespoons Lemon Juice~27g
1 teaspoon Black Pepper~2g
1/3 cup Ghee~93g
12 cups Water

Traditional Method of Preparation:

- In a cooking pan, combine meat, black pepper, and 12 cups of water. Cook over medium heat for 20 minutes until meat is tender
- In a saucepan, heat ghee and fry onions and French cut green beans over medium heat for 10 minutes
- Add tomatoes and continue frying for 5 minutes; stir constantly to prevent sticking
- Combine all ingredients together. Cover and cook over medium heat for 30 minutes.; stir occasionally
- Ready to serve

Healthy Recipe, 4 Servings, 4 Cups:

1 1/3 cups Steamed French Cut Green Beans~226g
3.2 oz. Lean Shank Meat~91.5g
1 cup Chopped Tomatoes~282g
3/4 cup Chopped Onions~113g
1 3/4 Tablespoons Lemon Juice~27g
1 teaspoon Black Pepper~2g
2 1/4 teaspoons Ground Flaxseed~5.6g
1/3 cup Tomato Juice~86g
4 cups Water

Healthy Method of Preparation:

- In a cooking pan, bring 4 cups of water to a boil, combine meat, black pepper and onion. Cook over medium heat for 20 minutes, until meat is tender
- Steam French cut green beans at high heat for 15 minutes (alternatively, mix 1 cup of water with 2 2/3 cups of French cut green beans and cook over medium heat, until beans are tender and water evaporates)
- Add tomato; lemon juice, tomato juice, and steamed French green beans to meat and onions; and cook over medium heat for 10 minutes
- Turn stove off; sprinkle ground flaxseed
- Ready to serve

Nutritional Goal

The purpose of modification is to reduce calories, to control fat content and improve its quality, and to enrich food with fiber and nutrients. Calorie content of the healthy recipe is reduced by more than 80% as compared to calorie content of the traditional recipe. In the healthy recipe, calories from macronutrients are well balanced due to omitting ghee, reducing meat, and increasing French cut green beans. Thus, saturated fat and cholesterol are reduced by more than 90% in the healthy recipe, when compared to their levels in the traditional recipe. A comparison between nutritional analysis of the traditional and the healthy recipes shows that the healthy recipe has greater values of different nutrients. Fiber content is increased by more than 85%, vitamin A and potassium are increased by more than 40%. There is a significant increase in levels of B-complex vitamins, more than 200%, in addition to an increase in levels of iron and zinc by more than 500%. Calcium content of the healthy recipe is as twice as the calcium content of the traditional recipe. Moreover, levels of magnesium and vitamin C are also increased by more than 200%the . The healthy recipe is highly recommended to individuals with constipation, diabetes, high lipid profiles, osteoporosis, post menopause, malnutrition, and excessive body weight.

Nutrient Content	Traditional Recipe	Healthy Recipe
Portion	1 cup	1 cup
Weight (g)	221	228
Kilocalories (kcal)	861	81.7
Protein (g)	1.2	5.8
Carbohydrate (g)	4.6	14
Fat (g)	95.5	1.5
Saturated Fat (g)	59	0.3
Monounsaturated Fat (g)	27.5	0.5
Polyunsaturated Fat (g)	3.6	0.5
Trans Fatty Acid (g)	0	0
Cholesterol (g)	245	7
Omega-6 Linoleic (g)	0.05	0.1
Omega-3 Linolenic (g)	0.002	0.3
Fiber (g)	1.5	2.9
Sugar (g)	2.4	5.6
Water (L)	0.3	13.3
Thiamin (mg)	0.02	0.1
Riboflavin (mg)	0.01	0.07
Niacin (mg)	0.25	1.6
Vitamin B6 (mg)	0.045	0.2
Vitamin B12 (mcg)	0.02	0.6
Folate (DFE) mcg	8.2	27
Vitamin C (mg)	8.6	40.5
Vitamin D (mcg)	0	0
Vitamin A (RAE) (mcg)	102.2	182
Vitamin E (mg)	2.8	0.34
Calcium (mg)	9.7	27
Iron (mg)	0.1	0.9
Magnesium (mg)	5.9	23.4
Potassium (mg)	116	375
Zinc (mg)	0.1	1.5
Sodium (mg)	3.8	17

Portion 1 Cup

Number of Exchanges

Traditional Recipe
1/3 non-starchy vegetable exchange
2 1/3 meat exchange (high fat)
3 2/3 fat exchange (saturated)

Healthy Recipe
1 non-starchy vegetable exchange
3/4 meat exchange (medium fat)
1/2 fat exchange (Omega-3-FA)

Calories from Macronutrients

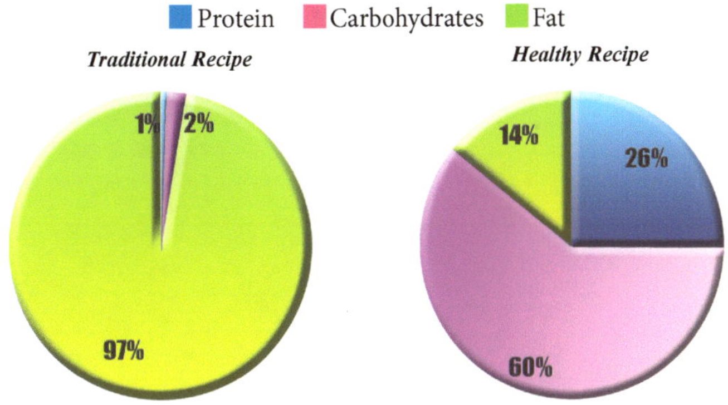

% Fiber Intake Compared to Average Daily Needs

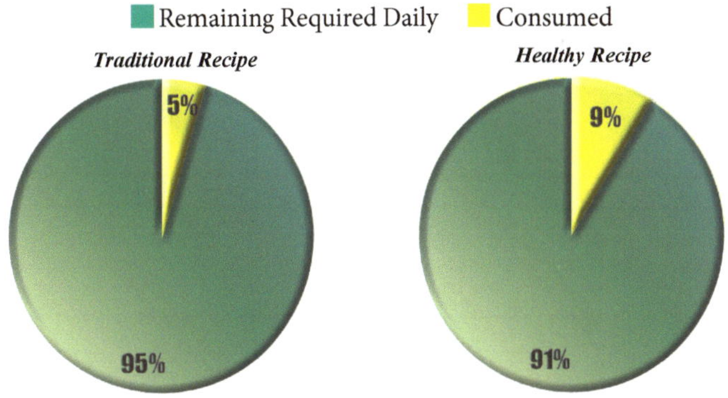

Recommended Portion Sizes & Meal Combinations

Traditional Recipe
(Calorie Controlled)

Men
1/2 cup of loubyah maraq
2/3 cup of traditional egg noodle rice

Women
1/3 cup of loubyah maraq
1/3 cup of traditional egg noodle rice

Healthy Recipe
(Calorie Controlled & Content Balanced)

Men
4 1/2 cups of loubyah maraq
3/4 cup of healthy egg noodle rice
(see page:128)
1 cup of lowfat ayran

Women
2 1/2 cups of loubyah maraq
1/2 cup of healthy egg noodle rice
(see page:128)
1 cup of lowfat ayran

Number of Exchanges in a Balanced Meal

Men
5 1/4 non-starchy vegetable exchange
3 1/4 meat exchange (medium fat)
3 1/2 fat exchange
(2 1/2 Omega-3-FA, 1 PUFA)
3 grain exchange
1 milk exchange

Women
3 non-starchy vegetable exchange
2 meat exchange (medium fat)
2 fat exchange
(1 1/3 Omega-3-FA, 3/4 PUFA)
2 grain exchange
1 milk exchange

French Green Beans Sautéed with Olive Oil & Cilantro

(Loubyah Bel-Zayet)

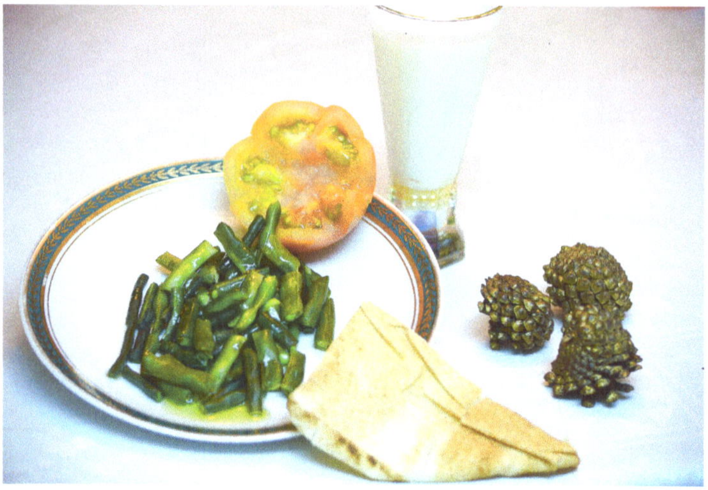

Traditional Recipe, 4 Servings, 4 Cups:

2 cups French Green Beans~491.4g
4 1/3 Tablespoons Fresh Chopped Cilantro~ 55.8g
2 1/3 Tablespoons Ground Garlic~28g
1/2 cup Olive Oil~111.6g
4 cups water

Healthy Recipe, 4 Servings, 4 Cups:

3 1/2 cup Steamed French Green Beans~603g
4 3/4 Tablespoons Fresh Chopped Cilantro~62.4g
1 3/4 Tablespoons Ground Garlic~20.8g
1 3/4 Tablespoons Olive Oil~23.4g
1/4 cup Lemon Juice~53g
1 cup water

Traditional Method of Preparation:

- In a cooking pan, heat olive oil and fry French green beans over medium heat for 5 minutes; stir frequently to prevent sticking
- Add 4 cups of water, cook over medium heat for another 15 minutes, until water evaporates
- Reduce heat, add cilantro and garlic, continue to cook over low heat for additional 5 minutes
- Ready to serve

Healthy Method of Preparation:

- In a steamer, place French green beans at high heat for 15 minutes until beans are tender. Alternatively, place beans with 1/2 cup of water and cook over medium heat for 15 minutes until water evaporates and beans are soft
- Add chopped cilantro to beans and continue steaming for another 5 minutes
- Transfer beans and cilantro to a cooking pan with 1/2 cup of water, lemon juice, and garlic. Cook over medium heat for 5 minutes, until water evaporates.
- Place food in shallow platter, drizzle with fresh olive oil
- Ready to serve

Nutritional Goal

The purpose of modification is to save calories, to improve quality of fat, and to add nutritional value. Calorie content of healthy recipe is reduced by half when compared to calorie content of traditional recipe. Although fat is still predominant in the healthy recipe, total fat and saturated fat are reduced by more than 70% when compared to their levels in the traditional recipe. The healthy method of preparation also preserves the nutrition quality of oil and prevents the transition of healthy fat into bad fat by heating the oil. A comparison between nutritional analysis of traditional and healthy recipes shows that the healthy recipe contains higher levels of different nutrients. Levels of thiamin and folate are increased by more than 20%, and levels of fiber, vitamin A, magnesium, and potassium are increased by more than 10%. The level of vitamin C is also increased by more than 100%. The healthy recipe is recommended to athletes and individuals with excess body weight, malnutrition, and post menopause. Following the recommended meal combination and portion sizes is important to balance the macronutrient contents of the entire meal.

Nutrient Content	Traditional Recipe	Healthy Recipe
Portion	1 cup	1 cup
Weight (g)	222	208
Kilocalories (kcal)	280.4	91
Protein (g)	1.8	2
Carbohydrate (g)	7	8.5
Fat (g)	28	5.9
Saturated Fat (g)	3.8	0.8
Monounsaturated Fat (g)	20.6	4.3
Polyunsaturated Fat (g)	2.8	0.6
Trans Fatty Acid (g)	0	0
Cholesterol (g)	0	0
Omega-6 Linoleic (g)	2.6	0.6
Omega-3 Linolenic (g)	0.2	0.04
Fiber (g)	2.5	3
Sugar (g)	2.4	3.2
Water (L)	0.017	0.03
Thiamin (mg)	0.03	0.04
Riboflavin (mg)	0.03	0.03
Niacin (mg)	0.2	0.2
Vitamin B6 (mg)	0.1	0.1
Vitamin B12 (mcg)	0	0
Folate (DFE) mcg	7.5	10
Vitamin C (mg)	3	8.6
Vitamin D (mcg)	0	0
Vitamin A (RAE) (mcg)	32	36.6
Vitamin E (mg)	3	0.8
Calcium (mg)	16.3	14
Iron (mg)	0.6	0.5
Magnesium (mg)	3.7	4.3
Potassium (mg)	56.6	69
Zinc (mg)	0.2	0.2
Sodium (mg)	2.3	1.5

Portion 1 Cup

Number of Exchanges

Traditional Recipe
2/3 non-starchy vegetable exchange
6 1/4 fat exchange (MUFA)

Healthy Recipe
2 non-starchy vegetable exchange
1 1/3 fat exchange (MUFA)

Calories from Macronutrients

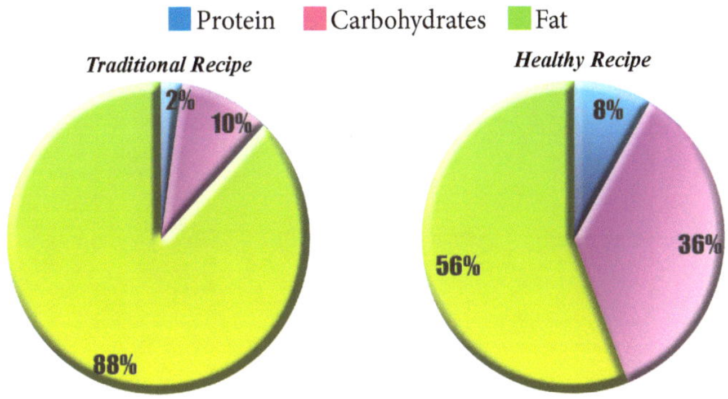

% Fiber Intake Compared to Average Daily Needs

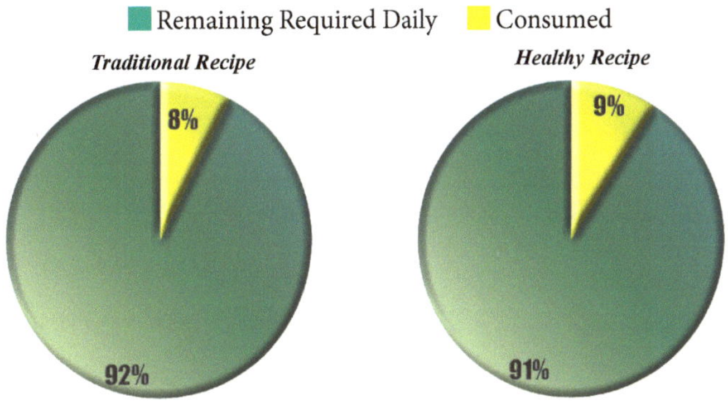

Recommended Portion Sizes & Meal Combinations

Traditional Recipe
(Calorie Controlled)

Men
2 1/4 cups of loubyah bel-zayet
2 slices of small white pita bread

Women
1 1/4 cups of loubyah bel-zayet
1 1/2 slices of small white pita bread

Healthy Recipe
(Calorie Controlled & Content Balanced)

Men
4 1/2 cups of loubyah bel-zayet
4 slices of small whole wheat pita bread
1 cup of lowfat ayran

Women
3 cups of loubyah bel-zayet
2 slices of small whole wheat pita bread
1 cup of lowfat ayran

Number of Exchanges in a Balanced Meal

Men
8 non-starchy vegetable exchange
6 fat exchange (MUFA)
4 grain exchange
1 milk exchange

Women
5 1/3 non-starchy vegetable exchange
4 fat exchange (MUFA)
2 grain exchange
1 milk exchange

Green Beans Stewed with Meat in Tomato Base

(Fasoleya'a Khadra'a Be Sous Al-Tamatum)

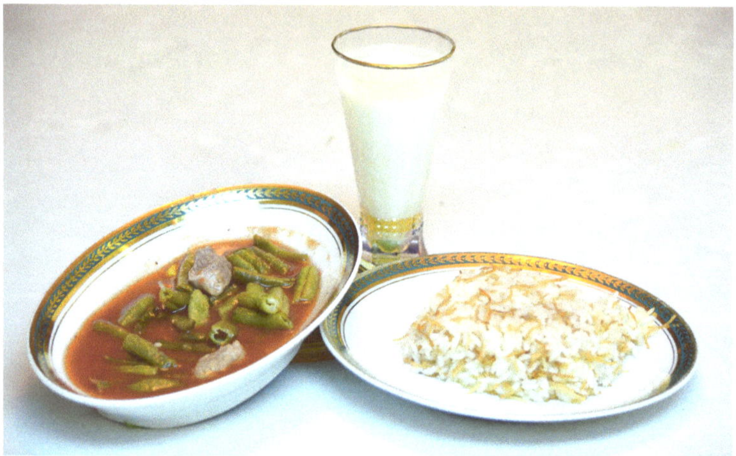

Traditional Recipe, 4 Servings, 4 Cups:

2 cups Fresh Green Beans~390.6g
2/3 cup Chopped Onions~105.4 g
6 1/2 Tablespoons Tomato Paste~101.68g
3.4 oz. Shank Meat~96.5g
1 teaspoon Black Pepper~2g
3 Tablespoons Corn Oil~42.16g
7 cups Water

Traditional Method of Preparation:

- Season meat with black pepper
- In a cooking pan, heat oil; fry chopped onions and meat over medium heat for 5-7 minutes, until meat is lightly brown
- Add beans and tomato paste and continue frying for 5 minutes; stir constantly to prevent sticking
- Combine all ingredients together with 7 cups of water
- Cook over medium heat for 30 minutes; stir occasionally
- Ready to serve

Healthy Recipe, 4 Servings, 4 Cups:

1 1/4 cups Fresh Green Beans~233.8g
1/3 cup Chopped Onions~48.7g
2/3 cup Tomato Paste~157.44 g
2.8 oz. Lean Shank Meat~80g
1 teaspoon Black Pepper~2g
2 1/2 teaspoons Flaxseed~6g
7 cups Water

Healthy Method of Preparation:

- Season meat with black pepper
- In a cooking pan, bring 7 cups of water to boil, combine meat and chopped onions. Cook over medium heat for 20 minutes
- Add beans and tomato paste, and continue to cook over medium heat for 10 minutes; stir thoroughly
- Turn stove off, add ground flaxseed, and stir twice
- Ready to serve

Nutritional Goal

The purpose of the modification aims to reduce calories and to balance calories from macronutrients. In order to balance the calories of macronutrient in the healthy recipe, fat and carbohydrates are reduced by more than 75% and 55% respectively, and protein is increased by more than 25%. A comparison between the traditional and healthy recipes shows that the calorie content of the healthy recipe is reduced by half when compared to the calorie content of the traditional recipe. Also, the total fat and saturated fat are reduced by more than 75% and 45% respectively, when omega-3-FA is increased by more than 170%. Although, fiber and nutrient contents of both recipes are approximately similar, following the recommended portion sizes and meal combination provides the body with great nutritional values. The healthy recipe is recommended to the elderly, athletes, dieters, and post-operative individuals.

Nutrient Content	Traditional Recipe	Healthy Recipe
Portion	1 cup	1 cup
Weight (g)	248	218
Kilocalories (kcal)	190	82.6
Protein (g)	7.6	10
Carbohydrate (g)	14.4	5.5
Fat (g)	12.45	2.4
Saturated Fat (g)	1.46	0.7
Monounsaturated Fat (g)	2.6	0.8
Polyunsaturated Fat (g)	6.3	0.6
Trans Fatty Acid (g)	0.03	0
Cholesterol (g)	0.77	13.6
Omega-6 Linoleic (g)	6.1	0.02
Omega-3 Linolenic (g)	0.13	0.37
Fiber (g)	4.8	2.24
Sugar (g)	5.6	1.3
Water (L)	15.4	25.7
Thiamin (mg)	0.13	0.1
Riboflavin (mg)	0.19	0.16
Niacin (mg)	2.7	3.2
Vitamin B6 (mg)	0.26	0.24
Vitamin B12 (mcg)	0.7	1.25
Folate (DFE) mcg	44	19.8
Vitamin C (mg)	23	3.2
Vitamin D (mcg)	0	0
Vitamin A (RAE) (mcg)	321	98.6
Vitamin E (mg)	3	0.1
Calcium (mg)	55	49.45
Iron (mg)	2.3	1.6
Magnesium (mg)	40.5	28.5
Potassium (mg)	580	304
Zinc (mg)	1.9	2.8
Sodium (mg)	220.8	425

Portion 1 Cup

Number of Exchanges

Traditional Recipe
1 non-starchy vegetable exchange
3/4 meat exchange (high fat)
2 1/4 fat exchange (PUFA)

Healthy Recipe
2/3 non-starchy vegetable exchange
2/3 meat exchange (medium fat)
2/3 fat exchange (Omega-3-FA)

Calories from Macronutrients

Protein Carbohydrates Fat

Traditional Recipe

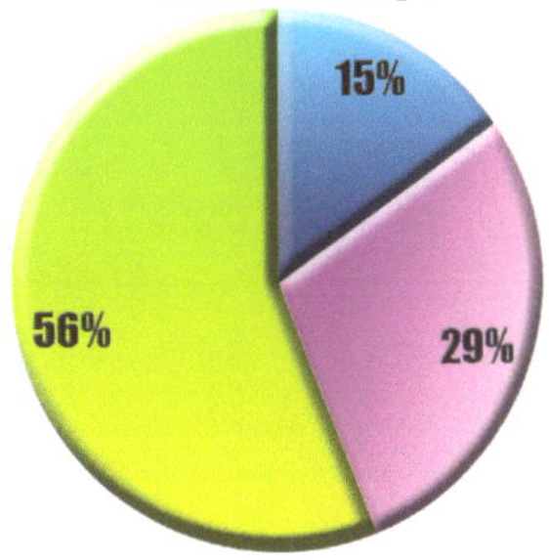

Healthy Recipe

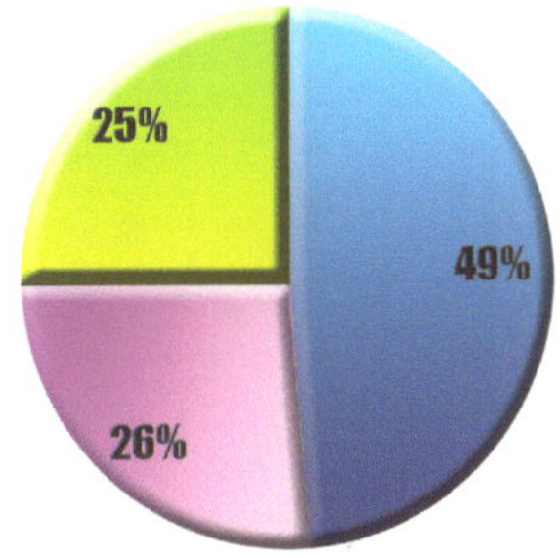

% Fiber Intake Compared to Average Daily Needs

Remaining Required Daily Consumed

Traditional Recipe

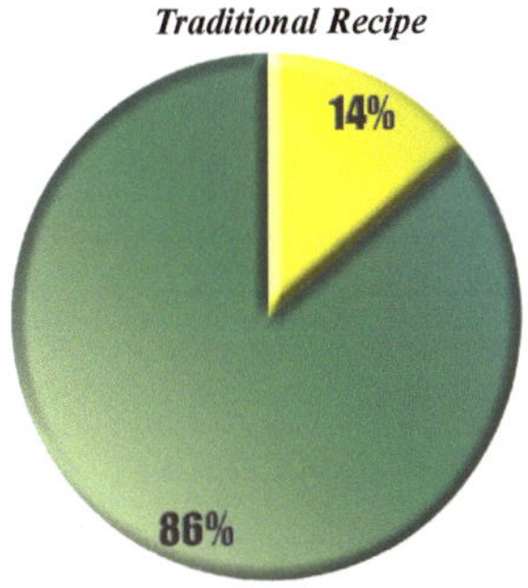

Healthy Recipe

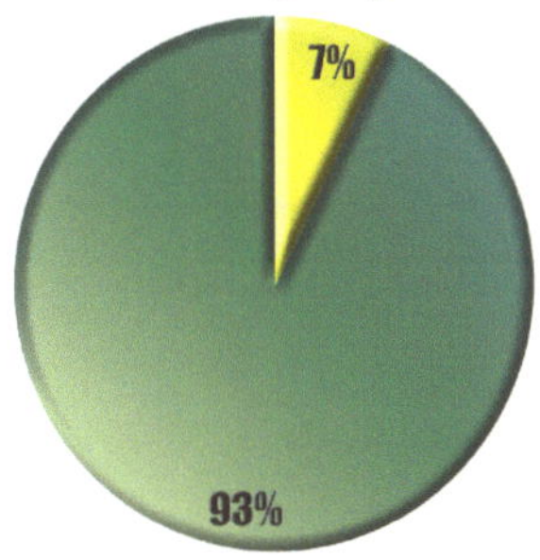

Recommended Portion Sizes & Meal Combinations

Traditional Recipe
(Calorie Controlled)

Men
1 1/4 cups of fasoleya'a khadra'a be sous al-tamatum
1 cup of traditional egg noodle rice

Women
1 cup of fasoleya'a khadra'a be sous al-tamatum
1/2 cup of traditional egg noodle rice

Healthy Recipe
(Calorie Controlled & Content Balanced)

Men
4 cups of fasoleya'a khadra'a be sous al-tamatum
3/4 cup of healthy egg noodle rice (see page:128)
1 1/2 cups of green salad-drizzled with vinegar
1 cup of lowfat ayran

Women
1 1/2 cups of fasoleya'a khadra'a be sous al-tamatum
1/2 cup of healthy egg noodle rice (see page:128)
1 1/2 cups of green salad-drizzled with vinegar
1 cup of lowfat ayran

Number of Exchanges in a Balanced Meal

Men
2 1/3 meat exchange (lean)
4 1/4 non-starchy vegetables exchange
3 1/2 fat exchange (2 1/3 Omega-3-FA, 1 PUFA)
3 grain exchange
1 milk exchange

Women
1 meat exchange (lean)
2 1/3 non-starchy vegetables exchange
1 3/4 fat exchange
(1 Omega-3-FA, 3/4 PUFA)
2 grain exchange
1 milk exchange

Green Beans Sautéed with Olive Oil & Cilantro

(Fasoleya'a Khadra'a Be Al-Zayet)

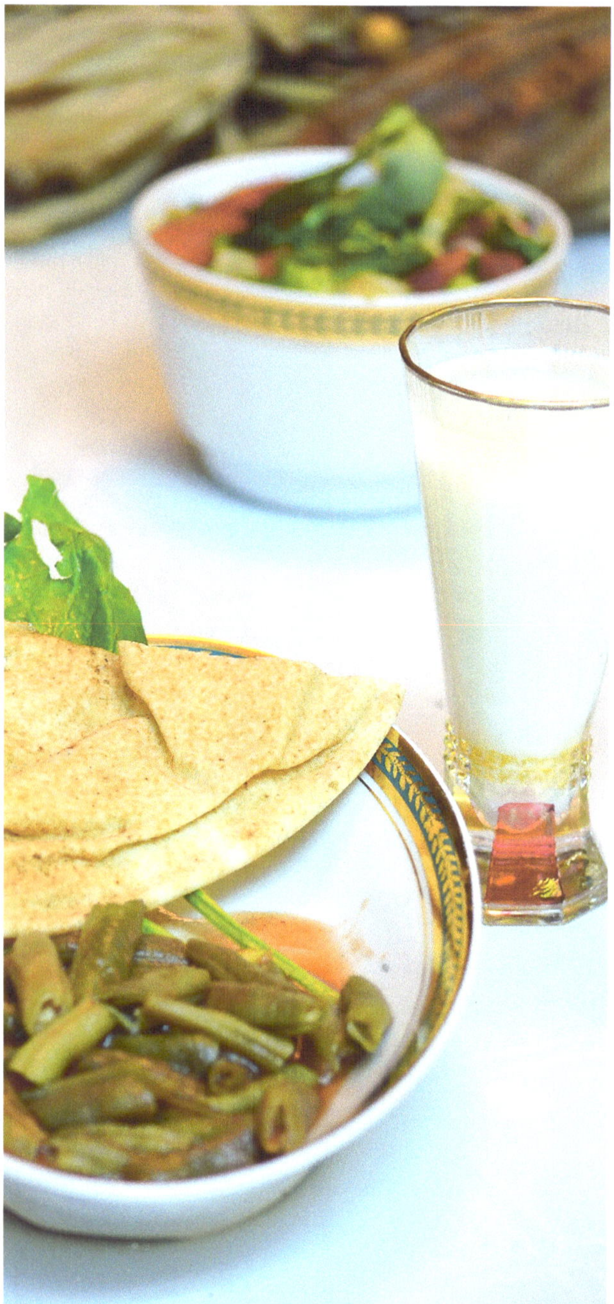

Traditional Recipe, 4 Servings, 4 Cups:

1 3/4 cups Fresh Green Beans~347.16g
1/2 cup Chopped Onions~91.08g
2 cups Diced Tomatoes~481.8g
1 1/3 teaspoons Ground Garlic~5.2g
1/3 cup Olive Oil~71.28g
2/3 teaspoon Chopped Cilantro~2.6g
3 cups Water

Traditional Method of Preparation:

- In a cooking pan, heat oil and fry onions and beans over medium heat for 5 minutes; stir frequently to prevent sticking
- Combine chopped tomatoes and 3 cups of water with beans; cook over medium heat for 15 minutes, until water evaporates
- Reduce heat, add cilantro and garlic; stir frequently for 2 minutes
- Ready to serve

Healthy Recipe, 4 Servings, 4 Cups:

1 1/2 cups Fresh Green Beans~290g
1/3 cup Chopped Onions~59.2g
2 3/4 cups Diced Tomatoes~674.88g
1 Tablespoon Ground Garlic~11.84g
1 Tablespoon Olive Oil~13g
1 1/3 teaspoons Chopped Cilantro~5.92g
1 cup Water

Healthy Method of Preparation:

- Steam green beans at high heat for 10 minutes. Alternatively, combine beans with onions and 5 cups of water
- Bring 1 cup of water to boil, add onions and steamed beans; cook over medium heat for 2 minutes
- Combine tomatoes and 1 cup of water with beans and onions; cook over medium heat for another 10 minutes, until water evaporates
- Reduce heat, add cilantro and ground garlic; stir frequently for 2 minutes
- Drizzle with olive oil
- Ready to serve

Nutritional Goal

The modification of this food is essential since the calories of the traditional recipe come mostly from fat. Also, the cooking method must be changed to preserve the quality of fat and to prevent the conversion of healthy fat into bad fat. The modification results in calorie reduction, higher quality of fat, fiber and micronutrient enrichments. The calories of the healthy recipe are reduced by more than half when compared to the calories of the traditional recipe. The nutritional analysis shows that the healthy recipe is enriched with more than 10% fiber, 90% folate, 120% magnesium, 30% iron, and 10% potassium, when compared to their levels in the traditional recipe. The healthy recipe is recommended to the elderly, children and individuals with appetite loss and constipation.

Nutrient Content	Traditional Recipe	Healthy Recipe
Portion	1 cup	1 cup
Weight (g)	198.6	234
Kilocalories (kcal)	217.1	90.6
Protein (g)	1.36	2.9
Carbohydrate (g)	12.37	13.7
Fat (g)	18.26	3.79
Saturated Fat (g)	2.48	0.56
Monounsaturated Fat (g)	13.36	2.5
Polyunsaturated Fat (g)	1.97	0.6
Trans Fatty Acid (g)	0	0
Cholesterol (g)	0	0
Omega-6 Linoleic (g)	1.8	0.56
Omega-3 Linolenic (g)	0.15	0.07
Fiber (g)	3.9	4.5
Sugar (g)	6.29	6
Water (L)	0.14	0.24
Thiamin (mg)	0.05	0.1
Riboflavin (mg)	0.06	0.1
Niacin (mg)	0.74	1.3
Vitamin B6 (mg)	0.13	0.24
Vitamin B12 (mcg)	0	0
Folate (DFE) mcg	22.6	45.5
Vitamin C (mg)	23.28	26.3
Vitamin D (mcg)	0	0
Vitamin A (RAE) (mcg)	435.76	550.9
Vitamin E (mg)	2.2	0.98
Calcium (mg)	59.8	61
Iron (mg)	0.87	1.22
Magnesium (mg)	15.7	38.27
Potassium (mg)	449.6	526.7
Zinc (mg)	0.24	0.7
Sodium (mg)	107.6	16

Portion 1 Cup

Number of Exchanges

Traditional Recipe
1 non-starchy vegetable exchange
4 fat exchange (MUFA)

Healthy Recipe
1 non-starchy vegetable exchange
3/4 fat exchange (MUFA)

Calories from Macronutrients

Protein Carbohydrates Fat

Traditional Recipe

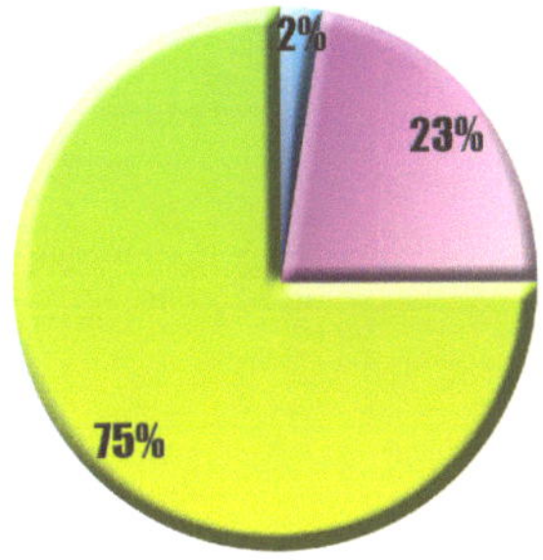

Healthy Recipe

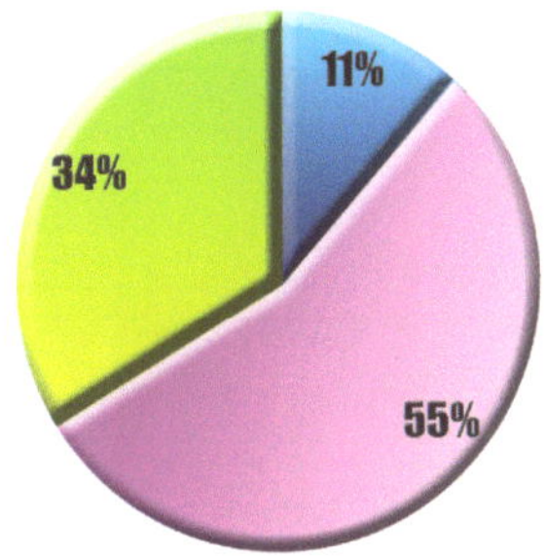

% Fiber Intake Compared to Average Daily Needs

Remaining Required Daily Consumed

Traditional Recipe

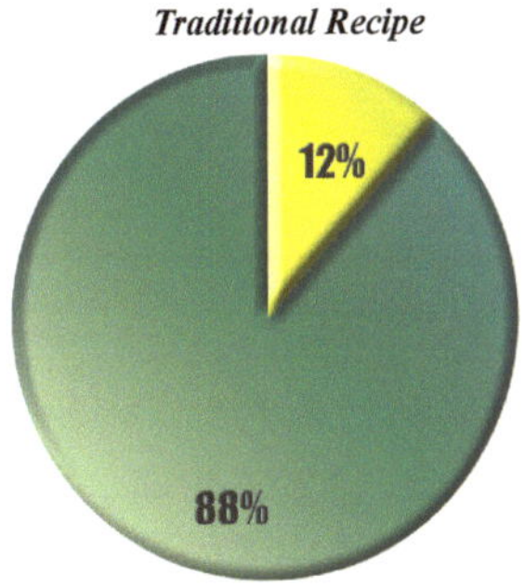

Healthy Recipe

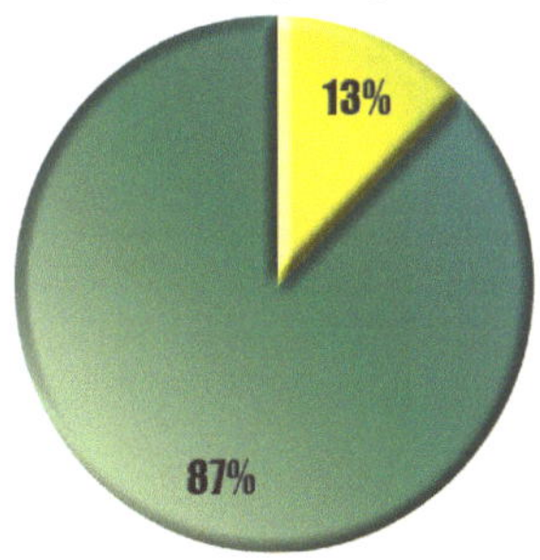

Recommended Portion Sizes & Meal Combinations

Traditional Recipe
(Calorie Controlled)

Men
2 1/2 cups of fasoleya'a khadra'a be al-zayet
3 slices of small white pita pread

Women
1 3/4 cups of fasoleya'a khadra'a be al-zayet
1 1/2 slices of small white pita pread

Healthy Recipe
(Calorie Controlled & Content Balanced)

Men
5 cups of fasoleya'a khadra'a be al-zayet
3 1/2 slices of small whole wheat pita pread
1 cup of lowfat ayran

Women
3 cups of fasoleya'a khadra'a be al-zayet
2 slices of small whole wheat pita pread
1 cup of lowfat ayran

Number of Exchanges in a Balanced Meal

Men
3 3/4 fat exchange (MUFA)
3 1/2 grain exchange
1 milk exchange
5 2/3 non-starchy vegetable exchange

Women
2 1/4 fat exchange (MUFA)
2 grain exchange
1 milk exchange
3 1/3 non-starchy vegetable exchange

Kidney Beans Stewed with Meat in Tomato Base

(Fasoleya'a Hab Be Sous Al-Tamatum)

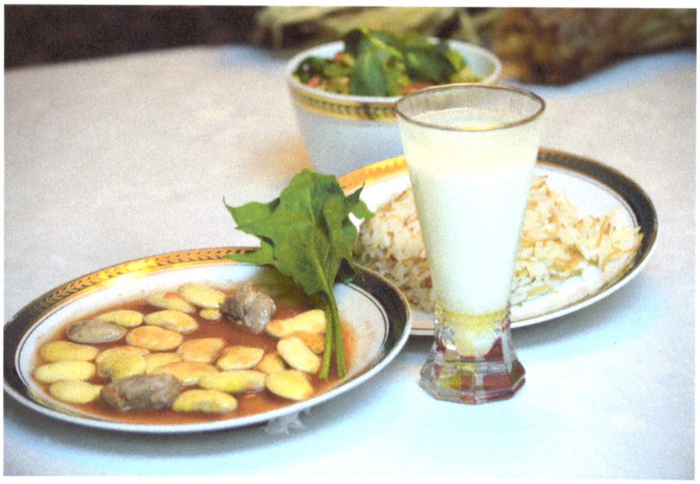

Traditional Recipe, 4 Servings, 4 Cups:

- 1 1/3 cups Kidney Beans~234.696g
- 3.6 oz. Shank Meat~102g
- 1/3 cup Tomato Paste~91.6g
- 1/3 cup Chopped Onion~55.88g
- 1 teaspoon Black Pepper~2g
- 1/3 cup Corn Oil~75.9g
- 9 cups Water

Traditional Method of Preparation:

- In a cooking pan, heat oil and fry chopped onions over medium heat for 5 minutes
- Season meat with black pepper, and combine it with onions. Continue to fry over medium heat for 8-10 minutes, until meat is lightly brown
- Add 9 cups of water and continue to cook over medium heat for 20 minutes
- Add beans and tomato paste to meat and onions, stir for 5 minutes
- Cook over medium heat for 40 minutes; stir occasionally
- Ready to serve

Healthy Recipe, 4 Servings, 4 Cups:

- 1 2/3 cups Kidney Beans~273g
- 4.6 oz. Broiled Lean Shank Meat~131g
- 1/2 cup Tomato Paste~141.7g
- 6 1/2 Tablespoons Chopped Onions~65g
- 1 teaspoon Black Pepper~2g
- 3 1/4 teaspoons Ground Flaxseed~8.125g
- 7 cups Water

Healthy Method of Preparation:

- Steam kidney beans on high heat for 30 minutes
- In a cooking pan, bring 7 cups of water to a boil then combine meat, tomato paste, and chopped onions
- Cook over medium heat for 20 minutes
- Add steamed beans, and continue to cook for another 5 minutes
- Turn stove off, add ground flaxseed; stir twice
- Ready to serve

Nutritional Goal

The modifications aim to reduce calories, to improve the quality of fat, and to enrich foods with nutrients. The calories of the healthy recipe are reduced by more than 40% when compared to the calories of the traditional recipe. Total fat and saturated fat are reduced by more than 75% in the healthy recipe, when compared to their levels in the traditional recipe. Also, cholesterol is reduced by half in the healthy recipe, when compared to the cholesterol level in the traditional recipe. The nutritional analysis of both recipes shows that the healthy recipe is enriched with different nutrients when compared to the traditional recipe. It has more than 25% fiber, 15% folate, 25% vitamin B12, 45% vitamin C, 50% vitamin A, 35% calcium, 30% iron, 30% magnesium, and 60% zinc. The healthy recipe is recommended to athletes and individuals with diabetes, anemia, osteoporosis, and constipation.

Nutrient Content	Traditional Recipe	Healthy Recipe
Portion	1 cup	1 cup
Weight (g)	248	260
Kilocalories (kcal)	339.5	182.8
Protein (g)	12.8	15
Carbohydrate (g)	20.8	26
Fat (g)	23.5	2.6
Saturated Fat (g)	4.6	0.7
Monounsaturated Fat (g)	6.26	0.8
Polyunsaturated Fat (g)	11.5	0.8
Trans Fatty Acid (g)	0.1	0
Cholesterol (g)	16.6	8.3
Omega-6 Linoleic (g)	11.2	0.13
Omega-3 Linolenic (g)	0.22	0.49
Fiber (g)	5.7	7.5
Sugar (g)	5.4	7.4
Water (L)	0.26	16
Thiamin (mg)	0.1	0.14
Riboflavin (mg)	0.2	0.19
Niacin (mg)	4	4.5
Vitamin B6 (mg)	0.2	0.3
Vitamin B12 (mcg)	0.7	0.9
Folate (DFE) mcg	99.4	118
Vitamin C (mg)	5.9	8.8
Vitamin D (mcg)	0	0
Vitamin A (RAE) (mcg)	106	163.7
Vitamin E (mg)	4	1.4
Calcium (mg)	42.6	59
Iron (mg)	2.7	3.6
Magnesium (mg)	56	74.9
Potassium (mg)	662	917.3
Zinc (mg)	1.5	2.5
Sodium (mg)	879	1093

Portion 1 Cup

Number of Exchanges

Traditional Recipe
2/3 starch exchange
1 2/3 meat exchange (2/3 very lean, high fat)
4 1/4 fat exchange (PUFA)
1/4 non-starchy vegetable exchange

Healthy Recipe
1 starch exchange
2 meat exchange (1very lean, 1 medium fat)
1 fat exchange (Omega-3-FA)
1/3 non-starchy vegetable exchange

Calories from Macronutrients

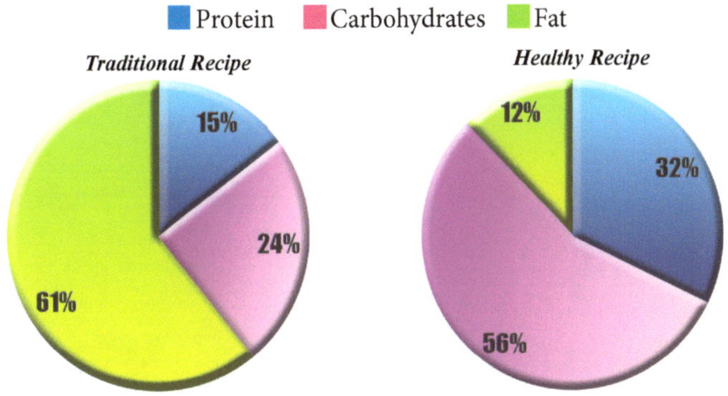

% Fiber Intake Compared to Average Daily Needs

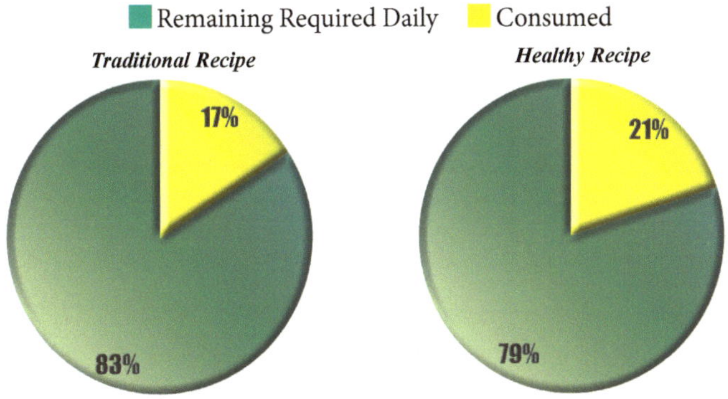

Recommended Portion Sizes & Meal Combinations

Traditional Recipe
(Calorie Controlled)

Men
1 cup of fasoleya'a hab be sous al-tamatum
3/4 cup of traditional egg noodle rice

Women
2/3 cup of fasoleya'a hab be sous al-tamatum
1/2 cup of traditional egg noodle rice

Healthy Recipe
(Calorie Controlled & Content Balanced)

Men
1 3/4 cups of fasoleya'a hab be sous al-tamatum
3/4 cup of healthy egg noodle rice (see page:128)
2 1/4 cups of green salad-drizzled with vinegar
1 cup of lowfat ayran

Women
1 cup of fasoleya'a hab be sous al-tamatum
1/3 cup of healthy egg noodle rice (see page:128)
2 cups of green salad-drizzled with vinegar
1 cup of lowfat ayran

Number of Exchanges in a Balanced Meal

Men
1 1/3 starch exchange
3 1/3 meat exchange (1 1/3 very lean, 2 medium fat)
3 non-starchy vegetable exchange
2 3/4 fat exchange(1 PUFA, 1 1/4 Omega-3-FA)
1 milk exchange
3 grain exchange

Women
1 starch exchange
2 meat exchange (1 very lean, 1 medium fat)
2 1/3 non-starchy vegetable exchange
1 1/2 fat exchange (1/2 PUFA, 1 Omega-3-FA)
1 milk exchange
1 1/4 grain exchange

Leek Cooked with Ground Meat & Cilantro

(Al-Korath Be Al-Lahem)

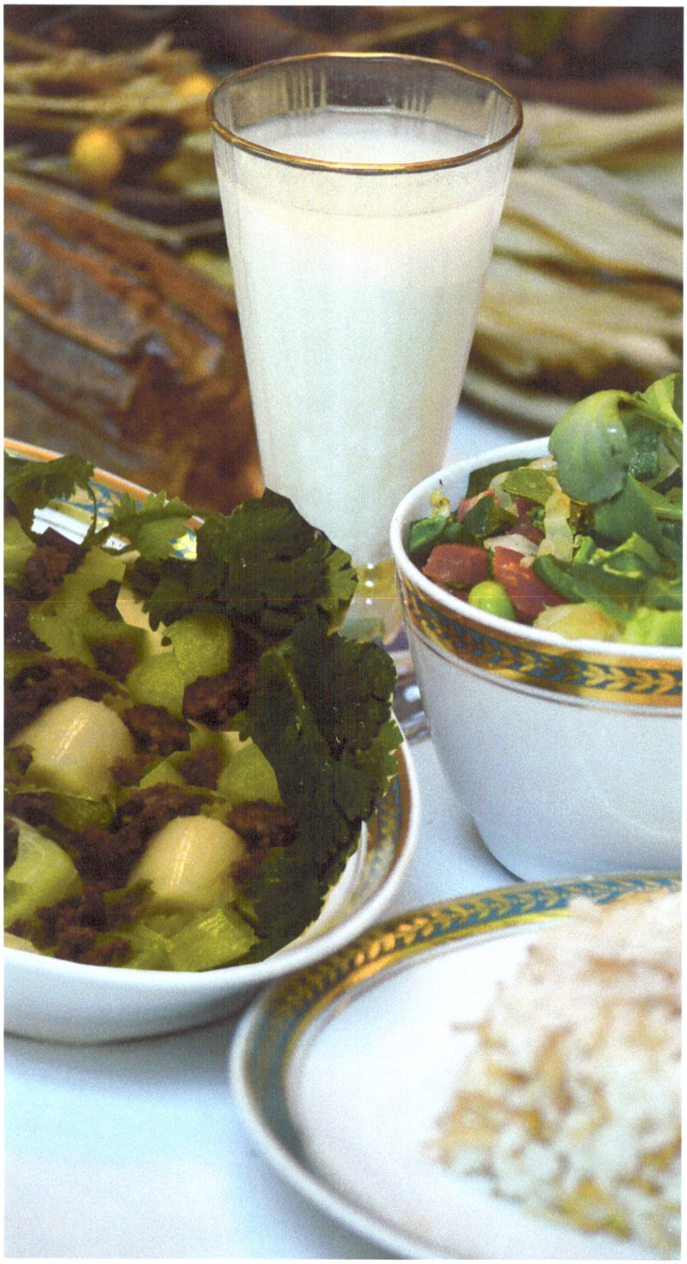

Traditional Recipe, 4 Servings, 4 Cups:

2 1/2 cups Fresh Chopped Leek~431.46g
4.4 oz. Medium Fat Ground Meat~124.8g
1/4 cup Fresh Chopped Cilantro~48.96g
9 1/4 Tablespoons Corn Oil~124.8g
1 teaspoon Black Pepper~2g

Traditional Method of Preparation:

- Season meat with black pepper
- Heat oil and fry meat over medium heat for 10 minutes until meat is brown
- Combine leek with meat; continue frying and stirring for 5 minutes
- Add cilantro to leek and meat; cover and cook over medium heat for 10 minutes; stir constantly to avoid sticking
- Turn stove off; set aside to settle for 5 minutes
- Ready to serve

Healthy Recipe, 4 Servings, 4 Cups:

4 3/4 cups Fresh Chopped Leek~818.7g
2.8 oz. Lean Meat~80g
2 Tablespoons Fresh Chopped Cilantro~24g
2 teaspoons Corn Oil~9g
2 teaspoons Black Pepper~4g
4 teaspoons Ground Flaxseed~10g
2 Tablespoons Lemon Juice~30.5g
1/2 cup Water

Healthy Method of Preparation:

- Steam leek at high heat for 20 minutes
- Season meat with black pepper; brown it in pre-heated nonstick skillet with 1/4 cup of water and 2 tablespoons of lemon juice over medium heat for 8 minutes; stir frequently to avoid sticking
- In a cooking pan, combine steamed leek, browned meat, and cilantro with ¼ cup of water
- Cook over medium heat for 10 minutes
- Turn stove off, sprinkle flaxseed and drizzle with corn oil
- Ready to serve

Nutritional Goal

The modification of the traditional recipe is essential since fat is the predominant macronutrient in this food. Modification aims to add multiple nutritional values to the food. Balance of macronutrients is achieved in the healthy recipe, and quality of fat is also improved. In the healthy recipe; total fat, saturated fat, and trans fatty acid are reduced by more than 70%, when cholesterol is reduced by half as well. The ratio of omega-6: omega-3 is reduced to 2:1 comparing to 50:1 of e traditional recipe. There is a great enrichment in fiber content; the healthy recipe contains more than 85% fiber when compared to fiber content of traditional recipe. The nutritional analysis shows that the healthy recipe is also enriched with women's supportive nutrients: (calcium, iron, magnesium, and potassium). Also, vitamin C, thiamin, and vitamin B6 are significantly increased in the healthy recipe. The previous factors make the healthy recipe a choice for postmenopausal women, elderly, children, and individuals with digestive problems, diabetes, high lipid profile, and heart disease.

Nutrient Content	Traditional Recipe	Healthy Recipe
Portion	1 cup	1 cup
Weight (g)	244.16	241
Kilocalories (kcal)	475.6	187.9
Protein (g)	11	7.9
Carbohydrate (g)	17	30
Fat (g)	41	5
Saturated Fat (g)	7	1
Monounsaturated Fat (g)	11	1.2
Polyunsaturated Fat (g)	20.3	2.4
Trans Fatty Acid (g)	0.5	0.1
Cholesterol (g)	32	12.4
Omega-6 Linoleic (g)	19.8	1.5
Omega-3 Linolenic (g)	0.4	0.8
Fiber (g)	2.5	4.6
Sugar (g)	4.6	8.1
Water (L)	12.8	5.88
Thiamin (mg)	0.11	0.2
Riboflavin (mg)	0.13	0.1
Niacin (mg)	2.8	2
Vitamin B6 (mg)	0.45	0.6
Vitamin B12 (mcg)	1	0.4
Folate (DFE) mcg	86	138
Vitamin C (mg)	17.77	26
Vitamin D (mcg)	0	0
Vitamin A (RAE) (mcg)	637.7	1053
Vitamin E (mg)	6.9	2
Calcium (mg)	85.4	135
Iron (mg)	3.7	5.2
Magnesium (mg)	44.8	74
Potassium (mg)	422.3	495
Zinc (mg)	2.3	1.4
Sodium (mg)	61	57.8

Portion 1 Cup

Number of Exchanges

Traditional Recipe
3/4 non-starchy vegetable exchange
7 fat exchange (PUFA)
1 meat exchange
(medium fat)

Healthy Recipe
1 1/4 non-starchy vegetable exchange
2/3 meat exchange (lean)
1 1/2 fat exchange
(1/2 PUFA, 1 Omega-3-FA)

Calories from Macronutrients

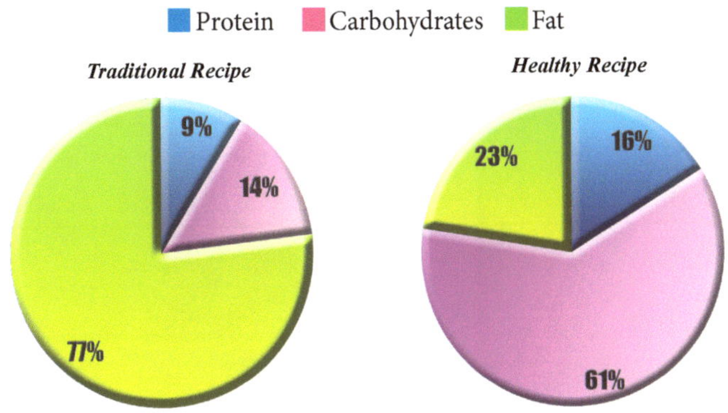

% Fiber Intake Compared to Average Daily Needs

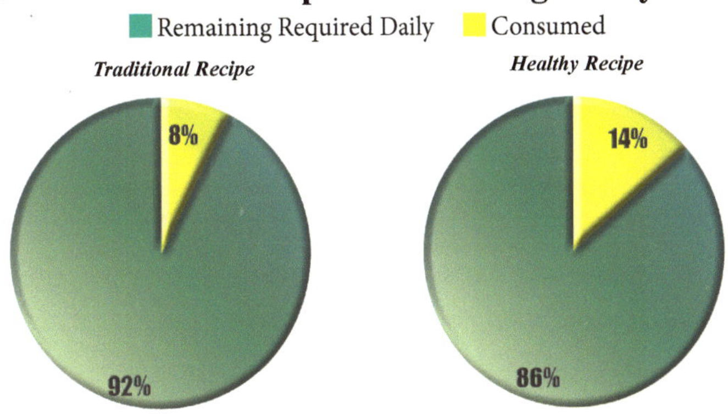

Recommended Portion Sizes & Meal Combinations

Traditional Recipe
(Calorie Controlled)

Men
1 cup of al-korath be al-lahem
1/2 cup of traditional egg noodle rice

Women
2/3 cup of al-korath be al-lahem
1/3 cup of traditional egg noodle rice

Healthy Recipe
(Calorie Controlled & Content Balanced)

Men
2 cups of al-korath be al-lahem
3/4 cup of healthy egg noodle rice
(see page:128)
1 cup of green salad-drizzled with vinegar
1 cup lowfat ayran

Women
1 1/4 cup of al-korath be al-lahem
1/3 cup of healthy egg noodle rice
(see page:128)
1 cup of green salad-drizzled with vinegar
1 cup lowfat ayran

Number of Exchanges in a Balanced Meal

Men
3 grain exchange
1 milk exchange
3 1/2 non-starchy vegetable exchange
1 1/3 meat exchange (lean)
4 fat exchange
(2 PUFA, 2 Omega-3-FA)

Women
1 1/4 grain exchange
1 milk exchange
2 2/3 non-starchy vegetable exchange
1 meat exchange (lean)
2 1/4 fat exchange
(1 PUFA, 1 1/4 Omega-3-FA)

Leek Sautéed with Olive Oil & Cilantro

(Al-Korath Be Al-Zeit)

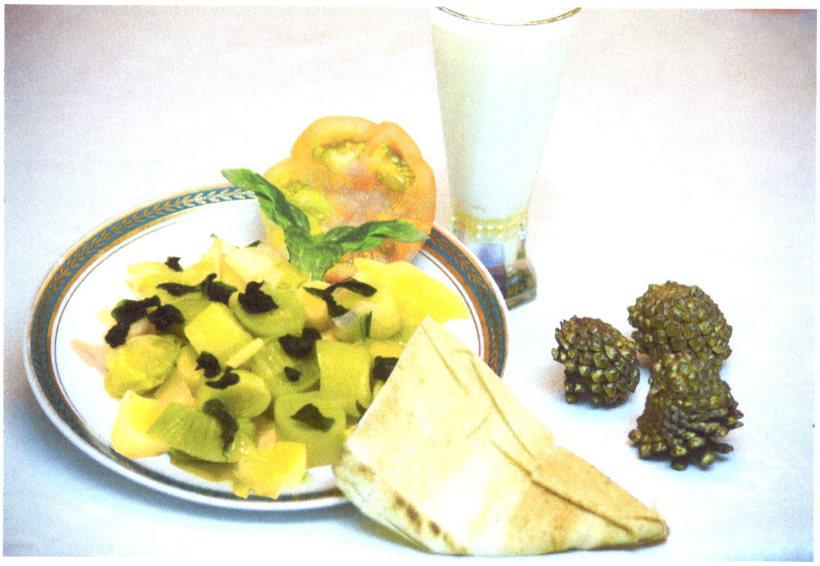

Traditional Recipe, 4 Servings, 4 Cups:

3 3/4 cups Fresh Chopped Leeks~632g
5 Tablespoons Fresh Chopped Cilantro~64g
1/2 cup Olive Oil~108g
3 cups Water

Traditional Method of Preparation:

- Heat oil in a cooking pan and fry leek over medium heat for 5 minutes
- Add 3 cups of water to pan and cook over medium heat for 15 minutes
- Add cilantro, stir continuously
- Cover and cook over medium heat for 3 minutes
- Remove the cover and reduce heat; cook for another 5 minutes over low heat
- Ready to serve

Healthy Recipe, 4 Servings, 4 Cups:

5 2/3 cups Fresh Chopped Leeks~949.5g
3 2/3 Tablespoons Chopped Fresh Cilantro~47.6g
3 1/2 teaspoons Olive Oil~15.3g
1/4 cup Water

Healthy Method of Preparation:

- Steam chopped leeks at high heat for 20 minutes, until leeks are tender
- In a cooking pan, combine leek and cilantro with 1/4 cup of water, and cook over medium heat for 5 minutes
- Turn stove off; drizzle with olive oil
- Ready to serve

Nutritional Goal

The modification of the recipe is essential since fat is the predominant macronutrient in the traditional recipe. The balance of calories from macronutrients results in many nutritional values added to the healthy recipe. The traditional cooking method, in which oil is heated, changes negatively the quality of fat in the body. The addition of olive oil at the end of cooking, as in the healthy recipe, preserves the quality and quantity of fat resulting in more pleasurable taste and great nutritious food. Thus, in the healthy recipe; saturated fat and total fat are reduced by more than 70%, and omega-6: omega-3 ratio is 2:1 in contrast to 7:1 of the traditional recipe. Also, the changes promote women's wellness since the healthy recipe is much richer with the nutrients women need. Calcium, folate, magnesium, zinc and iron are increased by more than 30%. Moreover, fiber content is more than 35% greater in the healthy recipe, when compared to fiber content of the traditional recipe. The modification and nutritional contents of the healthy recipe have positive health benefits to post-menopausal women, individuals with digestive problems, heart disease, and high lipid profiles.

Nutrient Content	Traditional Recipe	Healthy Recipe
Portion	1 cup	1 cup
Weight (g)	240	264
Kilocalories (kcal)	338.9	180.7
Protein (g)	2.7	3.8
Carbohydrate (g)	23	34
Fat (g)	27.5	4.6
Saturated Fat (g)	3.7	0.6
Monounsaturated Fat (g)	20	2.8
Polyunsaturated Fat (g)	3	0.8
Trans Fatty Acid (g)	0	0
Cholesterol (g)	0	0
Omega-6 Linoleic (g)	2.6	0.5
Omega-3 Linolenic (g)	0.37	0.26
Fiber (g)	3.3	4.6
Sugar (g)	6.3	9.4
Water (L)	15.5	11.2
Thiamin (mg)	0.11	0.15
Riboflavin (mg)	0.08	0.09
Niacin (mg)	0.8	1.07
Vitamin B6 (mg)	0.4	0.56
Vitamin B12 (mcg)	0	0
Folate (DFE) mcg	111	159.12
Vitamin C (mg)	23.45	31.7
Vitamin D (mcg)	0	0
Vitamin A (RAE) (mcg)	854	1238
Vitamin E (mg)	4.25	2.4
Calcium (mg)	104.6	148
Iron (mg)	3.8	5.2
Magnesium (mg)	48.5	69.5
Potassium (mg)	371	489
Zinc (mg)	0.27	0.34
Sodium (mg)	40	53

Portion 1 Cup

Number of Exchanges

Traditional Recipe
1 non-starchy vegetable exchange
6 fat exchange (MUFA)

Healthy Recipe
1 1/2 non-starchy vegetable exchange
1 fat exchange (MUFA)

Calories from Macronutrients

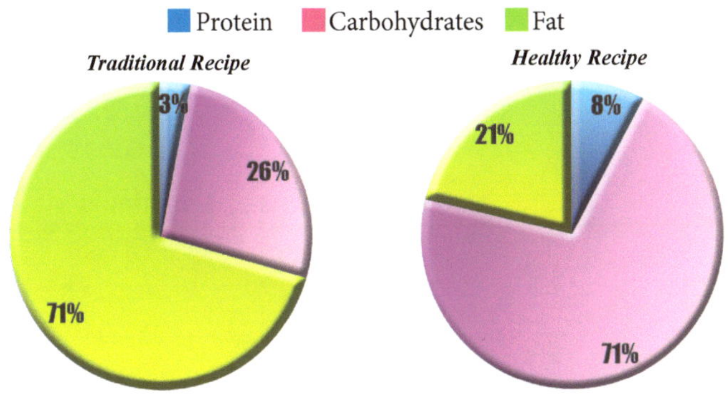

% Fiber Intake Compared to Average Daily Needs

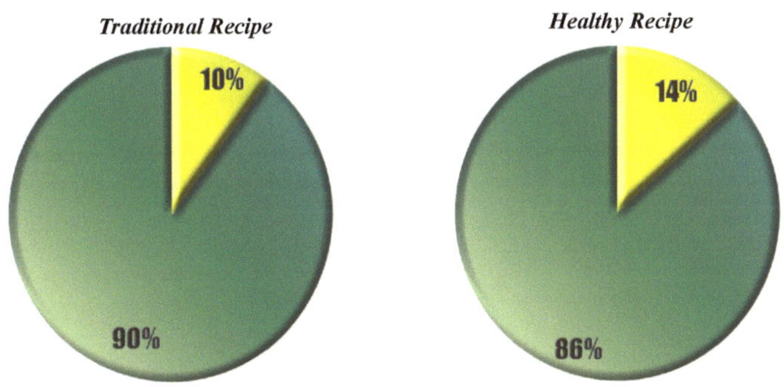

Recommended Portion Sizes & Meal Combinations

Traditional Recipe
(Calorie Controlled)

Men
2 cups of al-korath be al-zeit
1 1/2 slices of small white pita bread

Women
1 1/4 cups of al-korath be al-zeit
1 slice of small white pita bread

Healthy Recipe
(Calorie Controlled & Content Balanced)

Men
3 cups of al-korath be al-zeit
2 slices of small white pita bread
1 cup of lowfat ayran

Women
1 3/4 cup of al-korath be al-zeit
1 1/4 slices of small whole wheat pita bread
1 cup of lowfat ayran

Number of Exchanges in a Balanced Meal

Men
4 1/3 non-starchy vegetable exchange
2 1/2 fat exchange (MUFA)
1 milk exchange
2 grain exchange

Women
2 2/3 non-starchy vegetable exchange
1 1/2 fat exchange (MUFA)
1 milk exchange
1 1/4 grain exchange

Meat, Peas, and Carrots Stewed in Tomato Base

(Bazela'a wa Jazar Be Sous Al-Tamatum)

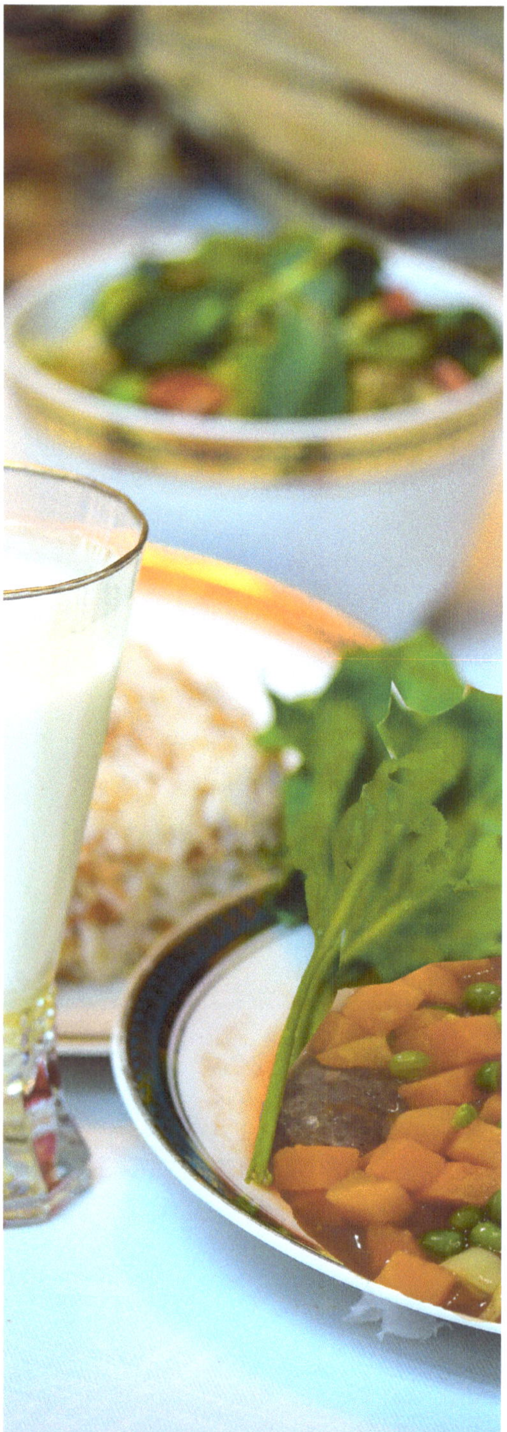

Traditional Recipe, 4 Servings, 4 Cups:

1 3/4 cups Diced Carrot~276g
1 cup Fresh Green Peas~180g
2/3 cup Chopped Onions~96g
2 1/2 Tablespoons Tomato Paste~40g
4 oz. Ground Meat~114g (Shank maybe used)
1 teaspoon Black Pepper~2g (Optional)
1 1/2 Tablespoons Corn Oil~20g
6 cups Water

Traditional Method of Preparation:

- In a cooking pan, heat oil and fry chopped onion over high heat for 5 minutes
- Season meat with black pepper and combine with onions, and continue frying for 5 minutes, until meat is brown
- Add peas and diced carrot; cook over medium heat for 5 minutes. Stir constantly to prevent sticking
- Add tomato paste and stir for another 2 minutes
- Add 6 cups of water, cook over medium heat for 20 minutes; stir occasionally
- Ready to serve

Healthy Recipe, 4 Servings, 4 Cups:

1 cup Diced Carrots~144.6g
1 cup Fresh Green Peas~173.54g
1/2 cup Chopped Onions~72.3g
1/2 cup Tomato Paste~118g
1.7 oz. Lean Ground Meat~48.8g (Lean Shank Meat maybe used)
1 teaspoon Black Pepper~2 g (Optional)
2/3 Tablespoon Ground Oatmeal~3.6g
1 teaspoon Ground Flaxseed~2.25g
5 cups Water

Healthy Method of Preparation:

- Steam green peas and carrot at high heat for 20 minutes
- Season meat with black pepper
- In a cooking pan, combine tomato paste, meat, onions, and 5 cups of water
- Cook over medium heat for 20 minutes; stir continuously, until meat is broiled and water is thicker and red
- Combine steamed vegetables and ground oatmeal with meat and onions; cook for another 5 minutes
- Turn stove off, add ground flaxseed; stir twice
- Ready to serve

Nutritional Goal

The purpose of the modification is to reduce calorie, to balance calories from macronutrients, to improve the quality of fat, and to enrich food with fiber and nutrients. The calories of the healthy recipe are reduced by more than 20% when compared to the calories of the traditional recipe. Macronutrients of the healthy recipe are more balanced than macronutrients of the traditional recipe. Fat quality and quantity of healthy recipe are improved when compared to fat quality and quantity of the traditional recipe. Total fat, saturated fat, and cholesterol are reduced by more than 70%, trans fatty acid is totally eliminated, and Omega-3-FA is increased by more than 100%. A comparison between nutrient contents of recipes shows that the healthy recipe is enriched with fiber, thiamin, riboflavin, niacin, vitamin B12, folate, calcium, iron, magnesium, potassium, zinc, and vitamin C, when compared to their levels in the traditional recipe. The healthy recipe is recommended to individuals with excessive body weight, osteoporosis, and heart disease.

Nutrient Content	Traditional Recipe	Healthy Recipe
Portion	1 cup	1 cup
Weight (g)	205.5	230.5
Kilocalories (kcal)	152.1	111.1
Protein (g)	5.9	6.7
Carbohydrate (g)	15	20.7
Fat (g)	8.1	1
Saturated Fat (g)	0.94	0.23
Monounsaturated Fat (g)	1.66	0.28
Polyunsaturated Fat (g)	4.1	0.38
Trans Fatty Acid (g)	0.02	0
Cholesterol (g)	0.49	3.7
Omega-6 Linoleic (g)	4	0.12
Omega-3 Linolenic (g)	0.1	0.15
Fiber (g)	4.5	5.3
Sugar (g)	7.6	8.7
Water (L)	9.9	7.6
Thiamin (mg)	0.15	0.18
Riboflavin (mg)	0.1	0.15
Niacin (mg)	2.34	2.7
Vitamin B6 (mg)	0.2	0.28
Vitamin B12 (mcg)	0.45	0.3
Folate (DFE) mcg	16.7	48.6
Vitamin C (mg)	9.6	16.8
Vitamin D (mcg)	0	0
Vitamin A (RAE) (mcg)	2597.8	1743.8
Vitamin E (mg)	1.7	1.23
Calcium (mg)	31.6	42.7
Iron (mg)	1.31	2.29
Magnesium (mg)	14.9	43.5
Potassium (mg)	426.1	589.2
Zinc (mg)	1.17	1.62
Sodium (mg)	217	270.4

Portion 1 Cup

Number of Exchanges

Traditional Recipe
2/3 non-starchy vegetable exchange
1 1/2 meat exchange (1/2 very lean, 1 high fat)
1/2 starch exchange
1 fat exchange (PUFA)

Healthy Recipe
2/3 non-starchy vegetable exchange
1 meat exchange (1/2 very lean, 1/3 lean)
1/2 starch exchange
1/4 fat exchange (Omega-3-FA)

Calories from Macronutrients

Protein Carbohydrates Fat

Traditional Recipe

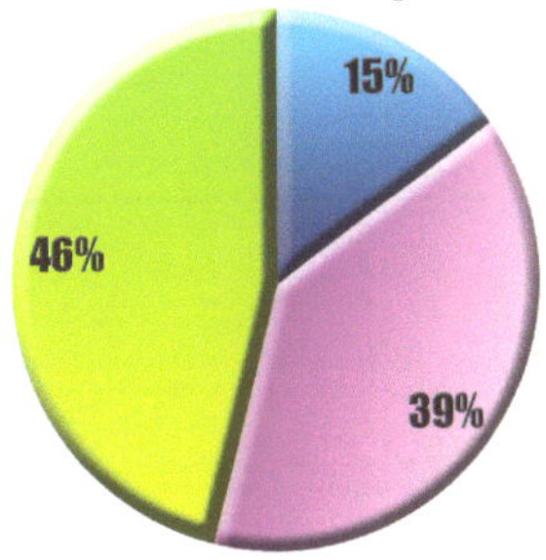

Healthy Recipe

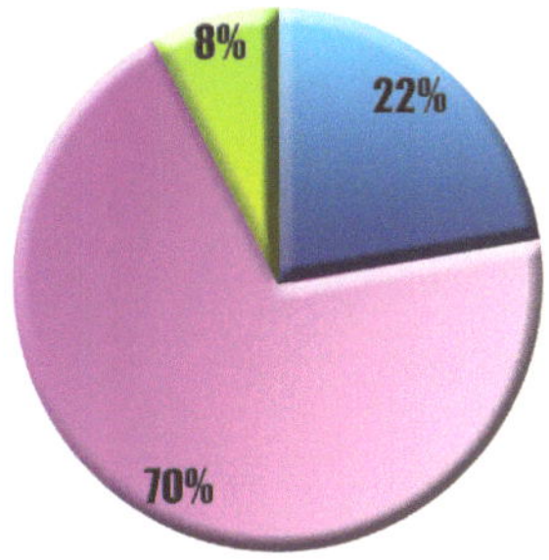

% Fiber Intake Compared to Average Daily Needs

Remaining Required Daily Consumed

Traditional Recipe

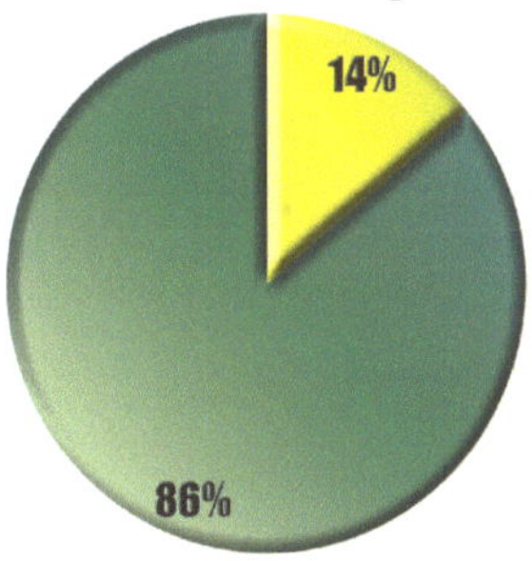

Healthy Recipe

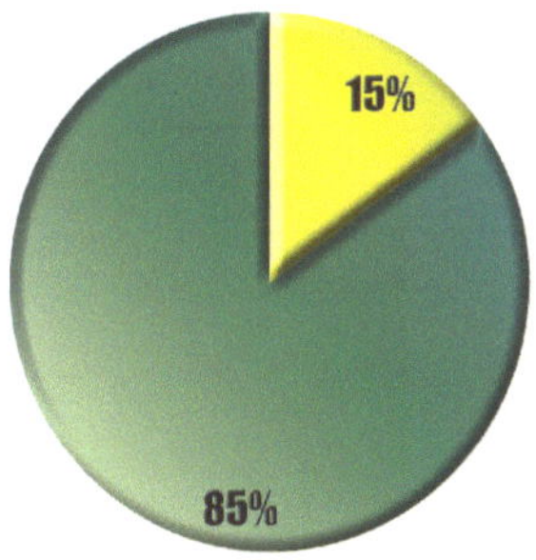

Recommended Portion Sizes & Meal Combinations

Traditional Recipe
(Calorie Controlled)

Men
2 1/2 cups of bazela'a wa jazar be Sous al-tamatum
3/4 cup of traditional egg noodle rice

Women
1 1/4 cups of bazela'a wa jazar be Sous al-tamatum
1/2 cup of traditional egg noodle rice

Healthy Recipe
(Calorie Controlled & Content Balanced)

Men
2 cups of bazela'a wa jazar be Sous al-tamatum
1 cup of healthy egg noodle rice (see page:128)
1 1/2 cups of green salad-drizzled with vinegar
1 cup of lowfat ayran

Women
1 1/2 cups of bazela'a wa jazar be Sous al-tamatum
1/2 cup of healthy egg noodle rice (see page:128)
1 cup of green salad-drizzled with vinegar
1 cup of lowfat ayran

Number of Exchanges in a Balanced Meal

Men
2 meat exchange (2/3 lean, 1 very lean)
3 non-starchy vegetable exchange
2 fat exchange (1 1/2 PUFA, 1/2 Omega-3-FA)
4 grain exchange
1 milk exchange
1 starch exchange

Women
1 1/4 meat exchange (1/2 lean, 3/4 very lean)
1 2/3 non-starchy vegetable exchange
1 fat exchange (3/4 PUFA, 1/3 Omega-3-FA)
2 grain exchange
1 milk exchange
3/4 starch exchange

Mushrooms Stewed with Ground Meat

(Mofarakah Be Al-Fotour)

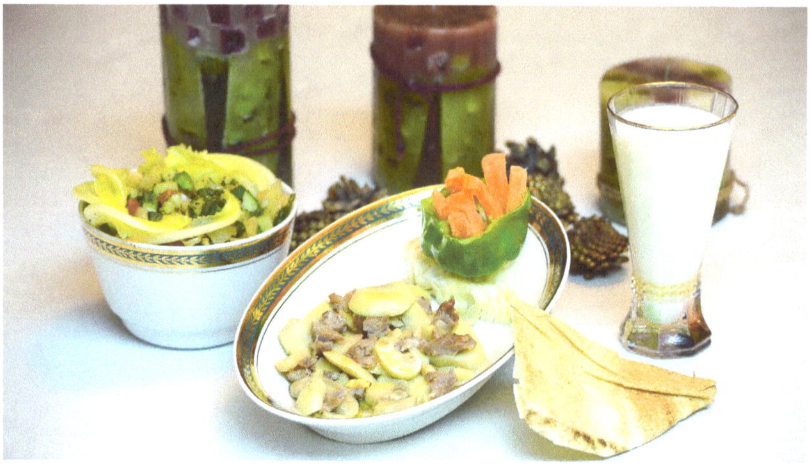

Traditional Recipe, 4 Servings, 4 Cups:

1 1/3 cups Sliced Mushroom~300g
1 1/3 cups Chopped Onions~217.6g
9.6 oz. Medium Fat Ground Meat~272g
3 1/4 Tablespoons Corn Oil~43.52g
4 teaspoons Black Pepper~8g
2 cups Water

Traditional Method of Preparation:

- Season meat with black pepper
- Wash and drain mushrooms
- In a cooking pan, heat oil and fry onions over medium heat for 5 minutes
- Combine meat with onions; continue cooking for 8-10 minutes, until meat is brown
- Add mushrooms; stir for 2 minutes
- Add 2 cups of water; cover and cook over medium heat for 20 minutes; stir occasionally to prevent sticking
- Ready to serve

Healthy Recipe, 4 Servings, 4 Cups:

2 cups Sliced Mushroom~448g
1 cup Chopped Onions~160g
4.2 oz. Lean Ground Meat~120g
4 teaspoons Corn Oil~18.4 g
4 teaspoons Black Pepper~8g
1/4 cup Lemon Juice~61g
4 teaspoons Flaxseed~10g
3 cups Water

Healthy Method of Preparation:

- Season meat with black pepper
- Wash and drain mushrooms
- In a cooking pan, broil meat in 2 cups of water over high heat for 10 minutes
- Add mushrooms and stir twice. Cover and cook over medium heat for 5 minutes
- In a saucepan, combine onions with 1 cup of water and bring to boil over medium heat for 10 minutes. Add olive oil and lemon juice then reduce to low heat; stir frequently for 30 seconds
- Combine sautéed onions and flaxseed with meat and mushrooms; stir frequently for 1 minute over low heat
- Ready to serve

Nutritional Goal

The purpose of this modification is to save calories, to reduce fat and sodium contents, and to enrich with fiber and nutrients. The calories of the healthy recipe are reduced by half when compared to calories of the traditional recipe. The healthy cooking method preserves the quality and quantity of fat. It prevents the conversion of healthy fat into bad fat by heating the oil. Total fat, saturated fat, cholesterol, and trans fatty acid are reduced by more than 60%, 70%, 50%, and 70% respectively. The nutritional analysis shows the healthy recipe is enriched with more than 45% fiber, and it contains more folate, vitamin C, vitamin A, and magnesium, when compared to the traditional recipe. The sodium content is also reduced by more than half in the healthy recipe. The healthy recipe is recommended to individuals with excessive body weight, malnutrition, folate-deficiency anemia, and constipation.

Nutrient Content	Traditional Recipe	Healthy Recipe
Portion	1 cup	1 cup
Weight (g)	173.2	222
Kilocalories (kcal)	286.2	144.2
Protein (g)	14.6	9.4
Carbohydrate (g)	9.9	12.13
Fat (g)	21.4	7.4
Saturated Fat (g)	5.4	1.4
Monounsaturated Fat (g)	7.12	1.9
Polyunsaturated Fat (g)	6.8	3.6
Trans Fatty Acid (g)	0.66	0.12
Cholesterol (g)	46.24	18.6
Omega-6 Linoleic (g)	6.6	2.8
Omega-3 Linolenic (g)	0.12	0.6
Fiber (g)	2.7	4
Sugar (g)	3.9	4.7
Water (L)	0.16	0.35
Thiamin (mg)	0.12	0.17
Riboflavin (mg)	0.13	0.1
Niacin (mg)	4.4	3.6
Vitamin B6 (mg)	0.36	0.27
Vitamin B12 (mcg)	1.47	0.67
Folate (DFE) mcg	23.44	27.22
Vitamin C (mg)	3.66	11.5
Vitamin D (mcg)	0	0
Vitamin A (RAE) (mcg)	0.8	1.4
Vitamin E (mg)	2.1	0.98
Calcium (mg)	35.32	31.5
Iron (mg)	2.4	1.8
Magnesium (mg)	30.66	38.36
Potassium (mg)	387.1	350
Zinc (mg)	3.7	2.5
Sodium (mg)	2227	497.8

Portion 1 Cup

Number of Exchanges

Traditional Recipe
2/3 non-starchy vegetable exchange
2 meat exchange (medium fat)
2 1/2 fat exchange (PUFA)

Healthy Recipe
1 non-starchy vegetable exchange
1 meat exchange (lean)
2 fat exchange
(1 PUFA,1 Omega-3-FA)

Calories from Macronutrients

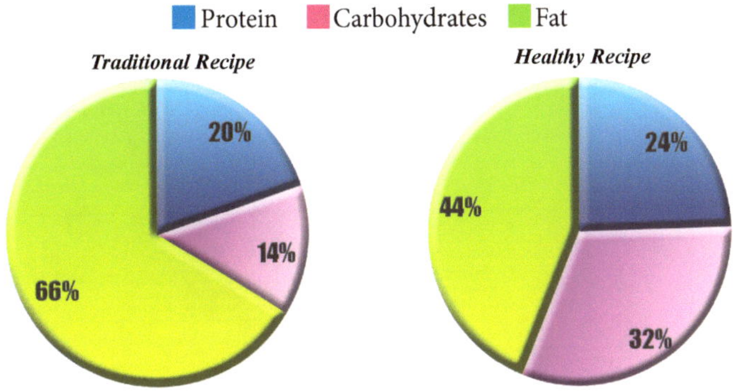

% Fiber Intake Compared to Average Daily Needs

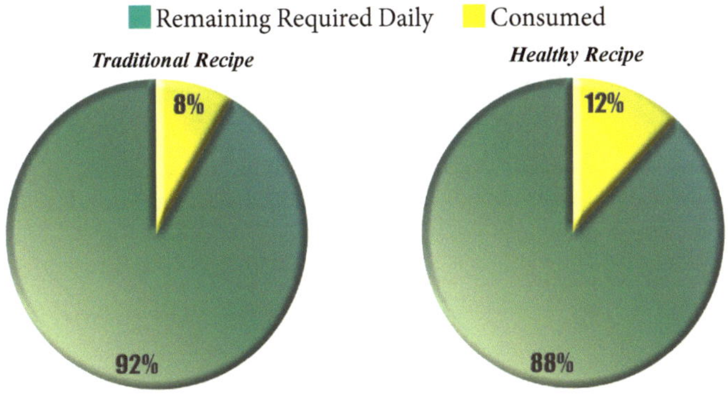

Recommended Portion Sizes & Meal Combinations

Traditional Recipe
(Calorie Controlled)

Men
1 3/4 cups of mofarakah be al-fotour
2 slices of small white pita bread
2/3 cup of regular plain yogurt

Women
1 cup of mofarakah be al-fotour
1 slice of small white pita bread
2/3 cup of regular plain yogurt

Healthy Recipe
(Calorie Controlled & Content Balanced)

Men
3 1/2 cups of mofarakah be al-fotour
2 1/2 slices of small whole wheat pita bread
2/3 cup of lowfat plain yogurt

Women
2 cups of mofarakah be al-fotour
1 1/2 slices of small whole wheat pita bread
2/3 cup of lowfat plain yogurt

Number of Exchanges in a Balanced Meal

Men
3 non-starchy vegetable exchange
7 fat exchange
(3 1/2 PUFA, 3 1/2 Omega-3-FA)
3 1/3 meat exchange (lean)
2 1/2 grain exchange
1 milk exchange

Women
1 1/4 non-starchy vegetable exchange
4 fat exchange (2 PUFA, 2 Omega-3-FA)
2 meat exchange (lean)
1 1/2 grain exchange
1 milk exchange

Mushrooms Stewed with Meat & Broth

(Foutour Be Maraq Al-Lahem)

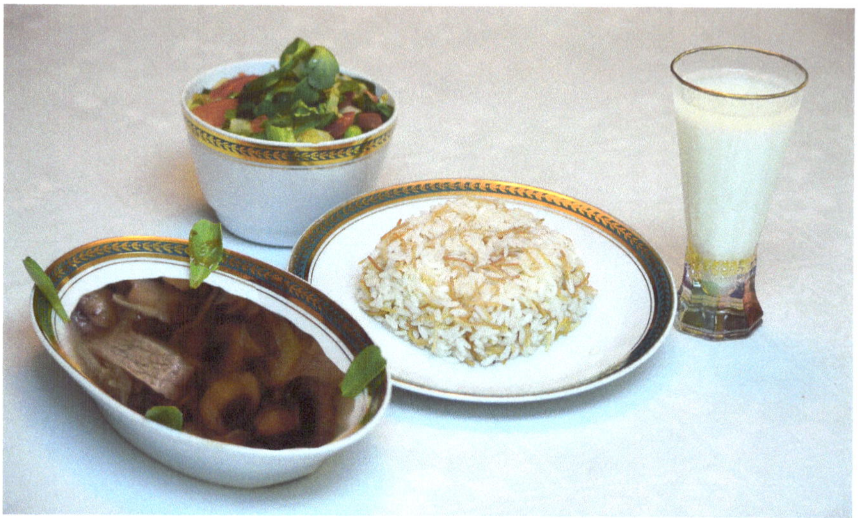

Traditional Recipe, 4 Servings, 4 Cups:

1 1/2 cups Sliced Onions~234.34g
1 1/4 cups Sliced Mushrooms~276g
4 oz. Shank Meat~114g (Ground Meat maybe used)
2 teaspoons Black Pepper~4g
7 cups Water

Traditional Method of Preparation:

- Combine onions, meat, black pepper, and 7 cups of water; cook over medium heat for 30 minutes
- Add mushrooms to pan, reduce heat; continue cooking for another 10 minutes
- Ready to serve

Healthy Recipe, 4 Servings, 4 Cups:

1 1/2 cups Sliced Onions~242.08g
1 1/2 cups Sliced Mushrooms~338.9g
2.7 oz. Lean Meat~78.6g
2 teaspoons Black Pepper~4g
1 Tablespoon Ground Flaxseed~7.5g
5 cups Water

Healthy Method of Preparation:

- Combine onions, meat, black pepper, and 5 cups of water; cook over medium heat for 20 minutes
- Add mushrooms to pan, reduce heat, and continue cooking for another 10 minutes
- Sprinkle flaxseed; stir twice
- Ready to serve

Nutritional Goal

The modifications aim to reduce calories, to balance calories from macronutrients, and to enrich foods with nutrients. The calorie content of the healthy recipe is reduced by more than 25% when compared to calorie content of the traditional recipe. Total fat and saturated fat are reduced by more than 60%, and trans fatty acid is totally eliminated. The addition of flaxseed increases the level of Omega-3-FA and leads to balance the ratio of omega-6: omega-3 in the healthy recipe. The nutritional analysis also demonstrates that the healthy recipe is enriched with more than 40% of fiber when compared to fiber content of the traditional recipe. The healthy recipe also has additional amount of women's supportive nutrients such as folate, calcium, and magnesium. The healthy recipe is recommended to individuals with diabetes, heart disease, high lipid profiles, constipation, and post menopause.

Nutrient Content	Traditional Recipe	Healthy Recipe
Portion	1 cup	1 cup
Weight (g)	144.8	223.9
Kilocalories (kcal)	104.7	80.55
Protein (g)	7.6	6.9
Carbohydrate (g)	8.6	10.17
Fat (g)	4.3	1.43
Saturated Fat (g)	1.7	0.24
Monounsaturated Fat (g)	1.88	0.36
Polyunsaturated Fat (g)	0.16	0.66
Trans Fatty Acid (g)	0.266	0
Cholesterol (g)	19.36	14.7
Omega-6 Linoleic (g)	0.107	0.06
Omega-3 Linolenic (g)	0.017	0.43
Fiber (g)	2	2.9
Sugar (g)	3.08	3.4
Water (L)	0.07	0.2
Thiamin (mg)	0.04	0.1
Riboflavin (mg)	0.05	0.1
Niacin (mg)	1.37	1.6
Vitamin B6 (mg)	0.186	0.2
Vitamin B12 (mcg)	0.617	0.27
Folate (DFE) mcg	12.83	16.1
Vitamin C (mg)	3.88	4
Vitamin D (mcg)	0	0
Vitamin A (RAE) (mcg)	0.73	1
Vitamin E (mg)	0.15	0.2
Calcium (mg)	20	26.7
Iron (mg)	1.1	0.9
Magnesium (mg)	12.2	19.6
Potassium (mg)	176.5	177.8
Zinc (mg)	1.37	1
Sodium (mg)	273.7	329.7

Portion 1 Cup

Number of Exchanges

Traditional Recipe
3/4 non-starchy vegetable exchange
1 meat exchange (medium fat)

Healthy Recipe
3/4 non-starchy vegetable exchange
2/3 meat exchange (lean)
3/4 fat exchange (Omega-3-FA)

Calories from Macronutrients

Protein Carbohydrates Fat

Traditional Recipe

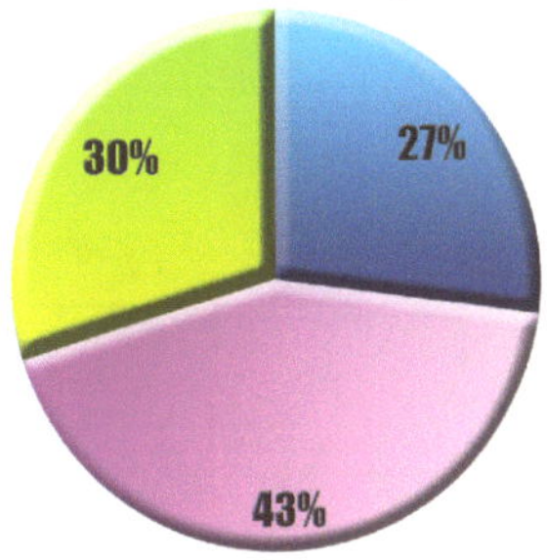

Healthy Recipe

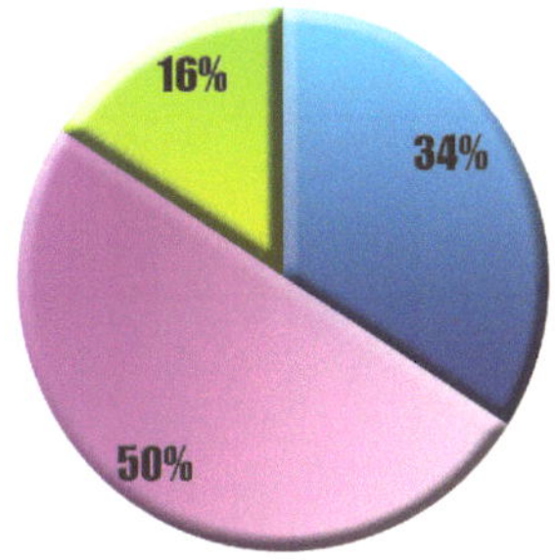

% Fiber Intake Compared to Average Daily Needs

Remaining Required Daily Consumed

Traditional Recipe

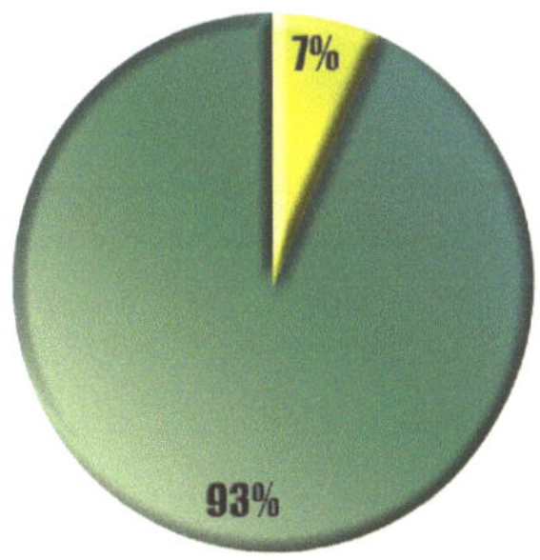

Healthy Recipe

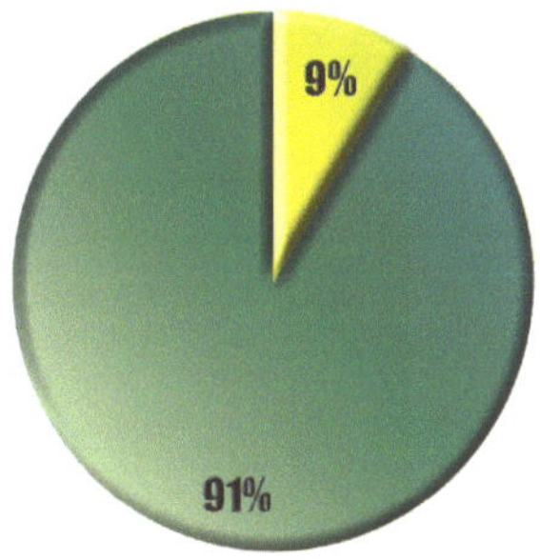

Recommended Portion Sizes & Meal Combinations

Traditional Recipe
(Calorie Controlled)

Men
3 cups of foutour be maraq al-lahem
1 cup of traditional egg noodle rice

Women
1 1/2 cups of foutour be maraq al-lahem
2/3 cup of traditional egg noodle rice

Healthy Recipe
(Calorie Controlled & Content Balanced)

Men
2 1/2 cups of foutour be maraq al-lahem
3/4 cup of healthy egg noodle rice (see page:128)
2 cups of green salad-drizzled with vinegar and olive oil
1 cup of lowfat ayran

Women
1 1/4 cups offoutour be maraq al-lahem
1/2 cup of healthy egg noodle rice (see page:128)
1 1/2 cups of green salad-drizzled with vinegar
1 cup of lowfat ayran

Number of Exchanges in a Balanced Meal

Men
3 3/4 non-starchy vegetable exchange
1 1/2 meat exchange (lean)
3 grain exchange
1 milk exchange
3 3/4 fat exchange (1PUFA, 1 MUFA, 2 Omega-3-FA)

Women
2 1/3 non-starchy vegetable exchange
1 meat exchange (lean)
2 grain exchange
1 milk exchange
1 3/4 fat exchange (3/4 PUFA, 1 Omega-3-FA)

Okra Cooked with Meat in Tomato Base

(Bamyah Bel Laham)

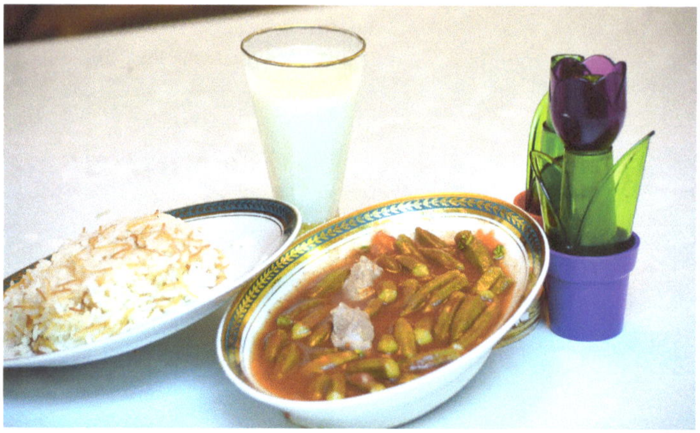

Traditional Recipe, 4 Servings, 4 Cups:

3.5 oz. Shank Meat~101g
1 1/2 Tablespoon Chopped Onions~23.6g
1 cup fresh Okra~104.9g
2 2/3 Tablespoon Corn Oil~35.9g
1/3 cup Tomato Paste~91.6g
7 cups Water

Traditional Method of Preparation:

- Bring 4 cups of water to boil; cook meat over medium heat for 20 minutes
- In a cooking pan, heat oil and fry chopped onions and okra over medium heat for 10 minutes
- Add tomato paste and continue frying for 5 minutes; stir constantly to prevent sticking
- Combine all ingredients together with 3 cups of water
- Cover and cook over medium heat for 30 minutes; stir occasionally
- Ready to serve

Healthy Recipe, 4 Servings, 4 Cups:

5.2 oz. Cooked Lean Shank Meat~149g
2/3 cup Chopped Onions~99.4g
1 3/4 cup Steamed Okra~305g
1 cup Tomato Juice~233g
2 2/3 cups Chopped Tomatoes~651g
1 3/4 Tablespoon Ground Flaxseed~13.7g
9 cups Water

Healthy Method of Preparation:

- Bring 6 cups of water to boil; cook meat over medium heat for 20 minutes
- Steam okra at high heat for 20 minutes
- Bring 3 cups of water to boil, combine okra, meat, meat broth, tomato juice, tomatoes and onions; cook over medium heat for 20 minutes
- Turn stove off, sprinkle ground flaxseed; stir twice
- Ready to serve

Nutritional Goal

The purpose of modification aims to reduce calories, to balance proportion of macronutrients, to improve fat quality, and to enrich food with fiber and nutrients. Calorie content of the healthy recipe is reduced by more than 10%, when compared to calorie content of the traditional recipe. Fat is the predominant macronutrient in the traditional recipe, when it is replaced with carbohydrate and protein in the healthy recipe. Thus, fat is reduced by more than 70%, when protein and carbohydrate are increased by more than 75% and 600% respectively. This is achieved by increasing the complex carbohydrate from okra and tomatoes. Quality of fat is also improved in the healthy recipe when compared to quality of fat in the traditional recipe. Saturated fat and cholesterol are reduced by more than 75% and 30% respectively, omega-6: omega-3 ratio is also improved when flaxseed is added. A comparison between nutritional analysis of the traditional and the healthy recipes shows that the healthy recipe contains greater levels of different nutrients. Thiamin and vitamin B6 content of thw healthy recipe are as twice as the traditional recipe. Riboflavin and vitamin B12 are increased by half, and niacin is increased by more than 25%. The healthy recipe is enriched with women's health nutrients as well. Folate, calcium, iron, magnesium, zinc and potassium are increased by more than 200%. Again, fiber is enriched by more than 500%, when sodium is reduced by more than 15%. The healthy recipe is recommended to different individuals with different chronic diseases including: (nervous illness, osteoporosis, diabetes, heart disease, malnutrition, constipation, and excessive body weight).

Nutrient Content	Traditional Recipe	Healthy Recipe
Portion	1 cup	1 cup
Weight (g)	212	228
Kilocalories (kcal)	144.14	125.9
Protein (g)	5.4	9.9
Carbohydrate (g)	2.4	17.7
Fat (g)	12.7	3
Saturated Fat (g)	3.1	0.6
Monounsaturated Fat (g)	3.6	0.9
Polyunsaturated Fat (g)	5.4	1.3
Trans Fatty Acid (g)	0.03	0
Cholesterol (g)	16.2	10
Omega-6 Linoleic (g)	5.2	0.3
Omega-3 Linolenic (g)	0.13	0.8
Fiber (g)	0.66	5
Sugar (g)	1	9.9
Water (L)	0.1	74.6
Thiamin (mg)	0.1	0.3
Riboflavin (mg)	0.13	0.2
Niacin (mg)	2.2	3.6
Vitamin B6 (mg)	0.1	0.4
Vitamin B12 (mcg)	0.6	0.9
Folate (DFE) mcg	40.2	164.4
Vitamin C (mg)	3.6	42.9
Vitamin D (mcg)	0	0
Vitamin A (RAE) (mcg)	28	509
Vitamin E (mg)	1.7	1.2
Calcium (mg)	29	106.5
Iron (mg)	0.62	2
Magnesium (mg)	16.7	78.4
Potassium (mg)	130.7	854
Zinc (mg)	0.9	2.8
Sodium (mg)	234.5	185.7

Portion 1 Cup

Number of Exchanges

Traditional Recipe
1 meat exchange (high fat)
2 fat exchange (PUFA)
1/3 non-starchy vegetable exchange

Healthy Recipe
1 1/3 meat exchange (medium fat)
1 1/3 fat exchange (Omega-3-FA)
2 non-starchy vegetable exchange

Calories from Macronutrients

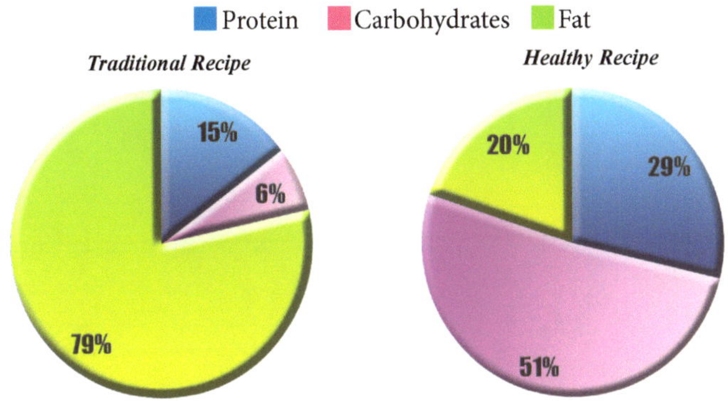

% Fiber Intake Compared to Average Daily Needs

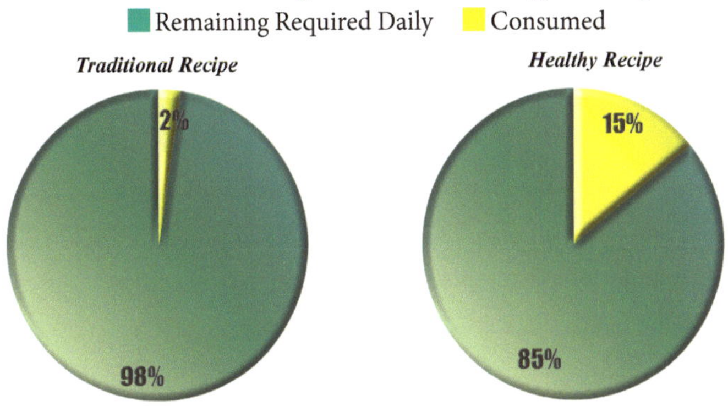

Recommended Portion Sizes & Meal Combinations

Traditional Recipe
(Calorie Controlled)

Men
2 1/2 cup of bamyah bel laham
3/4 cup of traditional egg noodle rice

Women
1 1/2 cup of bamyah bel laham
1/2 cup of traditional egg noodle rice

Healthy Recipe
(Calorie Controlled & Content Balanced)

Men
2 1/2 cup of bamyah bel laham
1 cup of healthy egg noodle rice
(see page:128)
1 cup of lowfat ayran

Women
1 1/4 cup of bamyah bel laham
2/3 cup of healthy egg noodle rice
(see page:128)
1 cup of lowfat ayran

Number of Exchanges in a Balanced Meal

Men
3 1/3 meat exchange (medium fat)
4 3/4 fat exchange (3 1/3 Omega-3-FA, 1 1/2 PUFA)
4 3/4 non-starchy vegetable exchange
4 grain exchange
1 milk exchange

Women
1 2/3 meat exchange (medium fat)
2 3/4 fat exchange (Omega-3-FA, 1 PUFA)
2 1/3 non-starchy vegetable exchange
2 1/2 grain exchange
1 milk exchange

Potatoes Stewed with Ground Meat

(Batata Be Al-Lahem)

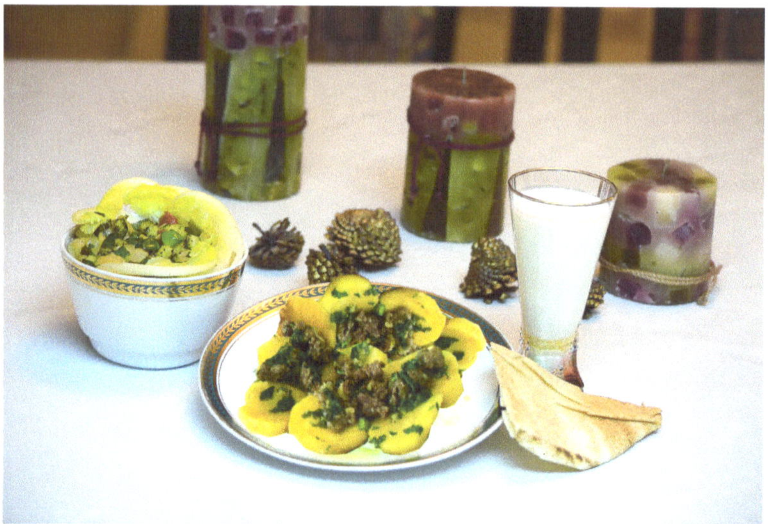

Traditional Recipe, 4 Servings, 4 Cups:

4 3/4 cups Diced Potatoes~1108g
10.5 oz. Ground Meat~298g
1 1/3 cups Chopped Onions~214g
1 1/2 teaspoons Black Pepper~3g
3 Tablespoons Corn Oil~40g
1 cup Water

Traditional Method of Preparation:

- Heat oil in large frying pan and fry potatoes over high heat for 10 minutes, until potatoes are gold
- Heat oil in a separate pan and gently fry onions for 10 minutes until onions are soft gold
- Season meat with black paper and add to onions
- Cook for another 10 minutes until meat is brown stirring frequently
- Add fried potatoes to onions and meat with 1 cup of water
- Cover and simmer over moderate heat for 10 minutes
- Ready to serve

Healthy Recipe, 4 Servings, 4 Cups:

3 cups Diced Potatoes~686.4g
6 oz. Lean Ground Meat~171.6g
3/4 cup Chopped Onions~132g
1 1/2 teaspoons Black Pepper~3g
4 1/2 Tablespoons Ground Flaxseed~33g
6 cups Water

Healthy Method of Preparation:

- Steam diced potatoes at high heat for 30 minutes until potatoes are very tender
- Season meat with black paper, add 6 cups of water and cook over medium heat for 20 minutes until meat is tender
- Combine onions with meat
- Cook for another 10 minutes over medium heat
- Add steamed potatoes to pan reduce heat and simmer gently on low heat for 2 minutes
- Remove from heat and sprinkle with flaxseed
- Ready to serve

Nutritional Goal

The purpose of modification is to reduce calories, to balance calories from macronutrients, and to enrich foods with nutrients. The calorie content of the healthy recipe is reduced by more than half when compared to the traditional recipe. Fat, protein, and carbohydrates are reduced by more than 80%, 20%, and 25% respectively. The healthy cooking method preserves the quality of fat; Omega-3-FA is increased by more than 300%, when saturated fat, cholesterol, and trans-fatty acid are reduced by more than 80%, 40%, and 75% respectively. The nutritional analysis also shows that the healthy recipe is enriched with more than 5% folate and magnesium when compared to the traditional recipe. The healthy recipe is recommended for to athletes and individuals with diabetes, malnutrition, and excessive body weight.

Nutrient Content	Traditional Recipe	Healthy Recipe
Portion	1 cup	1 cup
Weight (g)	248	245.85
Kilocalories (kcal)	697.58	251.43
Protein (g)	20.97	16
Carbohydrate (g)	49.15	33.5
Fat (g)	46.96	6
Saturated Fat (g)	8.8	1.4
Monounsaturated Fat (g)	13.4	1.6
Polyunsaturated Fat (g)	21.2	2.5
Trans Fatty Acid (g)	0.78	0.15
Cholesterol (g)	49.48	28.27
Omega-6 Linoleic (g)	20.86	0.02
Omega-3 Linolenic (g)	0.29	1.9
Fiber (g)	6	6
Sugar (g)	6.9	4.6
Water (L)	0.3	34.28
Thiamin (mg)	0.3	0.33
Riboflavin (mg)	0.197	0.14
Niacin (mg)	6.7	4.8
Vitamin B6 (mg)	0.8	0.57
Vitamin B12 (mcg)	1.58	1
Folate (DFE) mcg	14.25	15.7
Vitamin C (mg)	53.5	33.8
Vitamin D (mcg)	0	0
Vitamin A (RAE) (mcg)	1.9	1.2
Vitamin E (mg)	6.15	0.22
Calcium (mg)	59.56	55.9
Iron (mg)	4.7	3.55
Magnesium (mg)	81.28	85.5
Potassium (mg)	1654	1135
Zinc (mg)	4.14	3.3
Sodium (mg)	58.9	39.6

Portion 1 Cup

Number of Exchanges

Traditional Recipe
2 1/3 starchy vegetable exchange
2 1/4 fat exchange (PUFA)
2 1/3 meat exchange (medium fat)
1/3 non-starchy vegetable exchange

Healthy Recipe
1 1/2 starchy vegetable exchange
3 1/3 fat exchange (Omega-3-FA)
1 1/3 meat exchange (lean)

Calories from Macronutrients

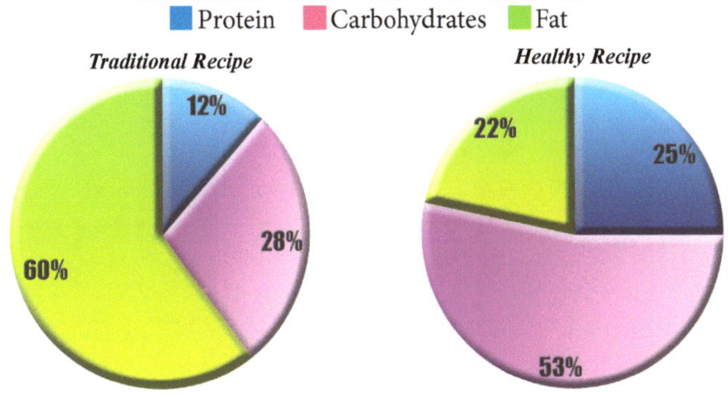

% Fiber Intake Compared to Average Daily Needs

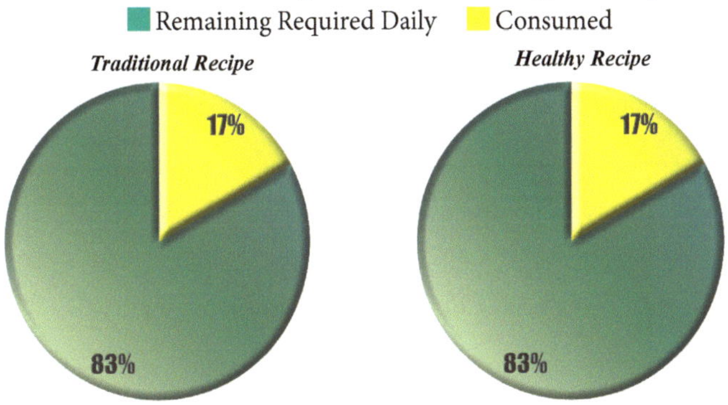

Recommended Portion Sizes & Meal Combinations

Traditional Recipe
(Calorie Controlled)

Men
1 cup of batata be al-lahem
1 slice of small white pita bread

Women
2/3 cup of batata be al-lahem
1/2 slice of small white pita bread

Healthy Recipe
(Calorie Controlled & Content Balanced)

Men
1 1/2 cups of batata be al-lahem
1 1/2 slices of small whole wheat pita bread
2 cups healthy green salad-drizzled with olive oil
1 cup lowfat ayran

Women
1 cup of batata be al-lahem
1 slice of small whole wheat pita bread
1cup of healthy green salad-drizzled with olive oil
1 cup of lowfat ayran

Number of Exchanges in a Balanced Meal

Men
2 1/4 starchy vegetable exchange
7 fat exchange (5 Omega-3-FA, 2 MUFA)
2 meat exchange (lean)
2 1/4 non-starchy vegetable exchange
1 1/2 grain exchange
1 milk exchange

Women
1 1/2 starchy vegetable exchange
4 1/3 fat exchange
(3 1/3 Omega-3-FA, 1 MUFA)
1 1/3 meat exchange (lean)
1 1/4 non-starchy vegetable exchange
1 grain exchange
1 milk exchange

Potatoes Stewed with Meat & Broth

(Al Batata Be Maraq Al-Lahem)

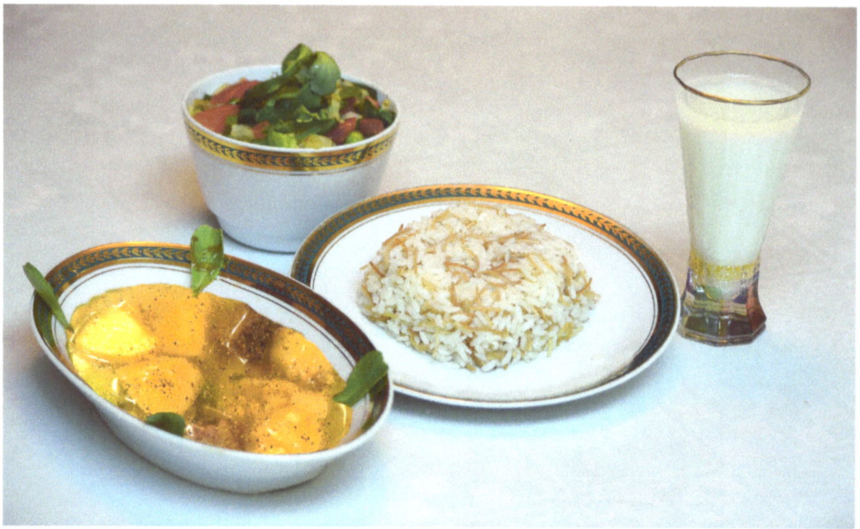

Traditional Recipe, 4 Servings, 4 Cups:

1 cup Diced Potatoes~255.5g
6.7 oz. Shank Meat~191.4g
1/3 cup Shredded Onions~58g
4 1/4 Tablespoons Corn Oil~58g
12 cups Water

Healthy Recipe, 4 Servings, 4 Cups:

1 1/4 cups Diced Boiled Potatoes~344g
2.3 oz. Lean Steak~66g
1 cup Chopped and Shredded Onions~160g
2 2/3 Tablespoons Ground Flaxseed~20g
10 cup Water

Traditional Method of Preparation:

- Bring 12 cups of water to boil, combine meat and onions and cook over medium heat for 25 minutes
- Heat oil and fry potatoes over medium heat for 10 minutes, until potatoes are gold
- Combine all ingredients and cook over medium heat for 10 minutes
- Ready to serve

Healthy Method of Preparation:

- Bring 10 cups of water to boil, combine meat and onions and cook over medium heat for 20 minutes
- Wash and boil potatoes with skin
- Peel potatoes and cut into medium-sized dices
- In a cooking pan, combine boiled potatoes, broiled meat, and onions; cook over medium heat for 20 minutes
- Turn stove off; sprinkle flaxseed
- Ready to serve

Nutritional Goal

The modification aims to reduce calories, to balance proportion of macronutrients, and to enrich food with fiber and nutrients. The calorie content of the healthy recipe is reduced by more than 35% when compared to calorie content of the traditional recipe. Fat is that predominant macronutrient in the traditional recipe, when it is reduced by more than 25% and replaced with more than 30% of carbohydrate in the healthy recipe. This change balances the calories from macronutrients and makes the healthy recipe a choice for individuals with diabetes. Also, the quality of fat is improved in the healthy recipe; total fat and saturated fat are reduced when Omega-3-FA is increased to balance the omega-6: omega-3 ratio. Fiber is increased by more than 150% in the healthy recipe, when compared to fiber content in the traditional recipe. Fiber enrichment helps individuals with digestive problems such as bloating and constipation. Scanning the nutrient contents of the healthy recipe, it contains more calcium, magnesium, folate, and iron, when compared to their levels in the traditional one. Thus, the nutritional values of the healthy recipe support women's health.

Nutrient Content	Traditional Recipe	Healthy Recipe
Portion	1 cup	1 cup
Weight (g)	232	264
Kilocalories (kcal)	274.9	164
Protein (g)	16.3	9.6
Carbohydrate (g)	14.3	22.8
Fat (g)	17	4.1
Saturated Fat (g)	2.7	0.96
Monounsaturated Fat (g)	4.9	1.2
Polyunsaturated Fat (g)	8.2	1.6
Trans Fatty Acid (g)	0	0
Cholesterol (g)	45.2	14.1
Omega-6 Linoleic (g)	0.17	0.03
Omega-3 Linolenic (g)	0.18	1.1
Fiber (g)	1.3	3.5
Sugar (g)	1	2.6
Water (L)	0.4	9.6
Thiamin (mg)	0.1	0.2
Riboflavin (mg)	0.2	0.12
Niacin (mg)	7.8	3.9
Vitamin B6 (mg)	0.5	0.36
Vitamin B12 (mcg)	1	0.5
Folate (DFE) mcg	18	23.3
Vitamin C (mg)	5.6	9
Vitamin D (mcg)	0	0
Vitamin A (RAE) (mcg)	0.7	1
Vitamin E (mg)	2.3	0.16
Calcium (mg)	38.3	43.5
Iron (mg)	1.2	1.3
Magnesium (mg)	32.8	49
Potassium (mg)	581.2	547.3
Zinc (mg)	2.6	1
Sodium (mg)	1027	739.5

Portion 1 Cup

Number of Exchanges

Traditional Recipe
1/2 starchy vegetable exchange
1 1/2 meat exchange (high fat)
3 exchange of fat exchange (PUFA)

Healthy Recipe
2/3 starchy vegetable exchange
1/2 meat exchange (lean)
2 fat exchange (Omega-3-FA)
1/4 non-starchy vegetable exchange

Calories from Macronutrients

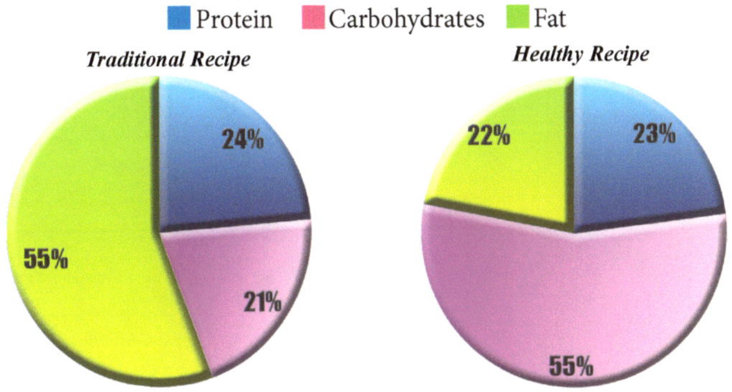

% Fiber Intake Compared to Average Daily Needs

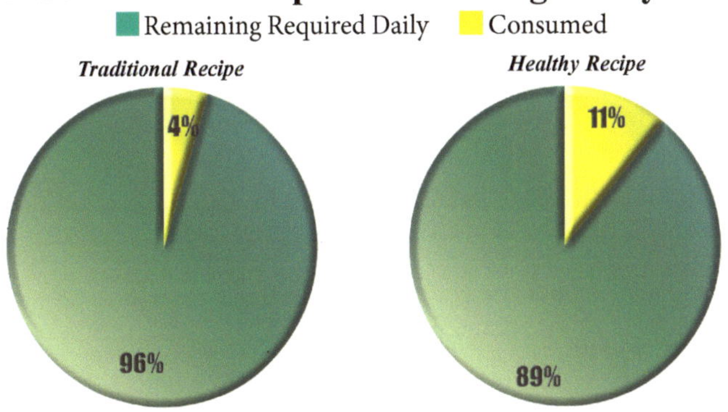

Recommended Portion Sizes & Meal Combinations

Traditional Recipe
(Calorie Controlled)

Men
1 1/4 cups of al batata be maraq al-lahem
3/4 cup of traditional egg noodle rice

Women
3/4 cup of al batata be maraq al-lahem
1/2 cup of traditional egg noodle rice

Healthy Recipe
(Calorie Controlled & Content Balanced)

Men
2 cups of al batata be maraq al-lahem
2/3 cup of healthy egg noodle rice
(see page:128)
3 cups of green salad-drizzled with vinegar
1 cup of lowfat ayran

Women
1 1/2 cups of al batata be maraq al-lahem
1/3 cup of healthy egg noodle rice
(see page:128)
1 1/2 cups of green salad-drizzled with vinegar
2/3 cup of lowfat ayran

Number of Exchanges in a Balanced Meal

Men
5 fat exchange (1 PUFA, 4 Omega-3-FA)
2 1/2 grain exchange
1 1/4 starchy vegetable exchange
3 1/4 non-starchy vegetable exchange
1 meat exchange (lean)
1 milk exchange

Women
3 1/2 fat exchange (1/2 PUFA, 3 Omega-3-FA)
1 1/4 grain exchange
1 starchy vegetable exchange
1 3/4 non-starchy vegetable exchange
3/4 meat exchange (lean)
2/3 milk exchange

Potato Sautéed with Olive Oil & Cilantro

(Batata Bel Al-Zeit wa Al-Kouzbara)

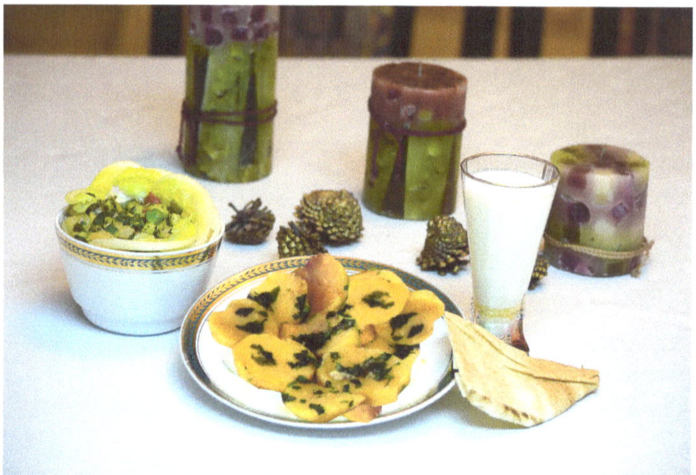

Traditional Recipe, 4 Servings, 4 Cups:

- 2 1/2 cups Diced Potatoes~584g
- 1 1/2 cups Chopped Onions~236g
- 9 Tablespoons Fresh Chopped Cilantro~116g
- 3 1/3 Tablespoons Ground Garlic~40g
- 1/4 cup Olive Oil~54.4g
- 4 cups Water

Traditional Method of Preparation:

- In a cooking pan, heat olive oil and fry onion over medium heat for 5 minutes
- Add diced potatoes, and continue frying until potatoes are gold
- Add 4 cups of water to pan; cover and cook over medium heat for 15-20 minutes, until water is absorbed; stir occasionally.
- Add garlic and cilantro to pan; stir twice
- Simmer for 5 minutes
- Ready to serve

Healthy Recipe, 4 Servings, 4 Cups:

- 2 cups Diced Potatoes~504.02g
- 1 1/3 cups Chopped Onions~217.25g
- 3 Tablespoons Fresh Chopped Cilantro~39.105g
- 2 teaspoons Ground Garlic~8.69g
- 2 teaspoons Olive Oil~9.7g
- 4 1/3 teaspoons Ground Flaxseed~10.8g
- 2 cups Water

Healthy Method of Preparation:

- Do not remove potatoes skin; wash and boil potato with the skin
- Peel potatoes and dice into medium size
- In a cooking pan, combine onions with 1 1/3 cups of water and bring to boil over medium heat for 12 minutes, until water evaporates and onions are thicker and juicy
- Combine boiled potatoes, garlic, and cilantro with onions; stir twice gently
- Add 2/3 cup of water, cover and cook over medium heat for another 5 minutes, until water evaporates
- Add flaxseed and simmer for 5 minutes
- Place food on a serving plate; sprinkle with fresh olive oil
- Ready to serve

Nutritional Goal

The purpose of the modification aims to reduce calorie and to improve the quality of fat. The calories provided by the healthy recipe are reduced by more than 15% when compared to the calories of the traditional recipe. The fat quantity of the healthy recipe is controlled resulting in reduction of more than 20% of total fat and 30% of saturated fat. The addition of flaxseed is the reason for an increase of more than 500% omega 3-FA. The cooking method of the healthy recipe preserves the quality of fat and saves the pleasurable taste of the food. Also, the sodium content of the healthy recipe is reduced by half, when compared to the sodium content of the traditional recipe. The healthy recipe is recommended to athletes, picky eaters, individuals with high blood pressure and excessive body weight.

Nutrient Content	Traditional Recipe	Healthy Recipe
Portion	1 cup	1 cup
Weight (g)	174	213.7
Kilocalories (kcal)	192	147.5
Protein (g)	5.4	4.1
Carbohydrate (g)	33	26.2
Fat (g)	5	3.3
Saturated Fat (g)	0.6	0.4
Monounsaturated Fat (g)	3.4	1.9
Polyunsaturated Fat (g)	0.5	0.7
Trans Fatty Acid (g)	0	0
Cholesterol (g)	0	0
Omega-6 Linoleic (g)	0.4	0.23
Omega-3 Linolenic (g)	0.04	0.33
Fiber (g)	4.5	3.7
Sugar (g)	5.4	4.6
Water (L)	26.9	9.2
Thiamin (mg)	0.2	0.18
Riboflavin (mg)	0.1	0.1
Niacin (mg)	2.2	1.7
Vitamin B6 (mg)	0.5	0.34
Vitamin B12 (mcg)	0	0
Folate (DFE) mcg	29.4	17.6
Vitamin C (mg)	41.2	29.4
Vitamin D (mcg)	0	0
Vitamin A (RAE) (mcg)	98.1	33.2
Vitamin E (mg)	1.3	0.6
Calcium (mg)	64	37.3
Iron (mg)	2	1.4
Magnesium (mg)	46.7	40
Potassium (mg)	986.6	756
Zinc (mg)	0.76	0.57
Sodium (mg)	21	10.7

Portion 1 Cup

Number of Exchanges

Traditional Recipe
1 1/4 starchy vegetable exchange
1/2 non-starchy vegetable exchange
3 fat exchange (MUFA)

Healthy Recipe
1 starchy vegetable exchange
1/3 non-starchy vegetable exchange
1 1/2 fat exchange (1/2 MUFA,
1 Omega-3-FA)

Calories from Macronutrients

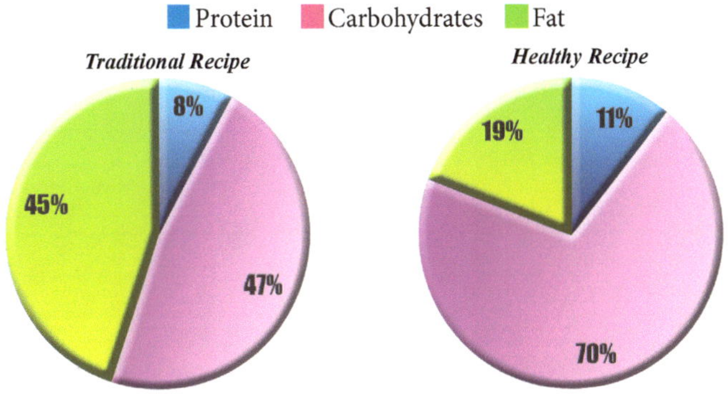

% Fiber Intake Compared to Average Daily Needs

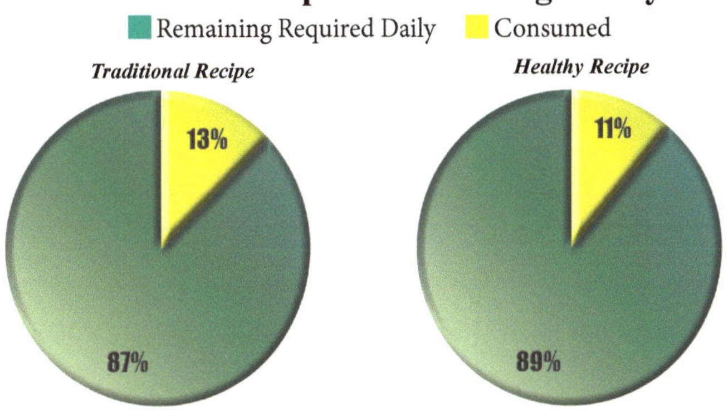

Recommended Portion Sizes & Meal Combinations

Traditional Recipe
(Calorie Controlled)

Men
2 1/2 cups of batata Be al-zeit wa al-kouzbara
2 1/2 slices of small white pita bread

Women
1 1/4 cups of batata Be al-zeit wa al-kouzbara
1 1/2 slices of small white pita bread

Healthy Recipe
(Calorie Controlled & Content Balanced)

Men
3 cups of batata Be al-zeit wa al-kouzbara
2 slices of small whole wheat pita bread
2 1/2 cups of green salad-drizzled with vinegar
1 cup of lowfat ayran

Women
1 3/4 cups of batata Be al-zeit wa al-kouzbara
1 slice of small whole wheat pita bread
1 1/2 cups of green salad-drizzled with vinegar
1 cup of lowfat ayran

Number of Exchanges in a Balanced Meal

Men
2 grain exchange
3 2/3 non-starchy vegetable exchange
4 1/2 fat exchange (1 1/2MUFA, 3 Omega-3-FA)
1 milk exchange
3 starchy vegetable exchange

Women
1 grain exchange
2 non-starchy vegetable exchange
2 3/4 fat exchange (1 MUFA, 1 3/4 Omega-3-FA)
1 milk exchange
1 3/4 starchy vegetable exchange

Potatoes Stewed with Tomatoes
(Mahmous)

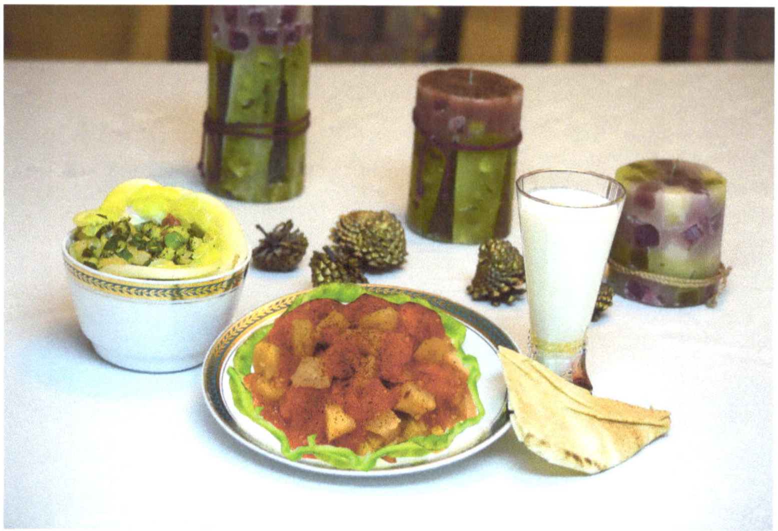

Traditional Recipe, 4 Servings, 4 Cups:

2 cups Diced Boiled Potatoes~470g
1 1/4 cups Diced Tomatoes~313.46g
1 3/4 cups Chopped Onions~274.28g
1 1/2 Tablespoons Ground Garlic~19g
6 1/2 Tablespoons Corn Oil~88.16g
3 3/4 cups Water

Traditional Method of Preparation:

- Cover potatoes with water and bring it to a boil for 20 minutes until potatoes are tender
- Heat oil and fry onions over medium heat for 4 minutes until onions are golden brown
- Combine tomato and garlic with onions and cook; stirring frequently for 5 minutes
- Add boiled potatoes and 3 3/4 cups of water to vegetables; cook over medium heat for 15 minutes
- Turn stove off, cover and allow to sit for 5 minutes
- Ready to serve

Healthy Recipe, 4 Servings, 4 Cups:

1 1/4 cups Diced Boiled Potatoes~259.5g
1 1/2 cups Diced Tomatoes~359g
2 1/2 cups Chopped Onions~399g
2 1/2 teaspoons Ground Garlic~10g
4 teaspoons Ground Flaxseed~10g
4 1/2 cups Water

Healthy Method of Preparation:

- Wash potatoes with skin; then boil potatoes with skin
- Peel potatoes and cut into medium sized dices
- In a deep cooking pan add onions with 2 1/2 cups of water and bring to a boil over medium heat for 15 minutes until water evaporates and onions are thick and juicy
- Combine tomatoes and garlic with onions and cook over moderate heat for 5 minutes
- Add boiled potatoes and 2 cups of water to vegetables, cover and cook for another 10 minutes until water evaporates
- Turn stove off, add flaxseed and allow to sit for 5 minutes
- Ready to serve

Nutritional Goal

The modification aims to reduce calories, to balance calories from macronutrients, and to enrich food with fiber and nutrients. Calorie content of the healthy recipe is reduced by more than half when compared to calorie content of the traditional recipe. The proportion of macronutrients is more balanced in the healthy recipe; carbohydrates and protein are replaced for fat. In the healthy recipe, total fat and saturated fat are also reduced by more than 85%, when compared to their levels in the traditional recipe. A comparison between nutrient contents of the healthy recipe and the traditional recipe shows that the healthy recipe contains more fiber, folate, vitamin A, vitamin E, calcium, magnesium, and iron. The healthy recipe is recommended to individuals with heart disease, osteoporosis, post menopause and excessive body weight.

Nutrient Content	Traditional Recipe	Healthy Recipe
Portion	1 cup	1 cup
Weight (g)	239.9	231.98
Kilocalories (kcal)	353.9	137.4
Protein (g)	3.8	3.7
Carbohydrate (g)	36.9	29.8
Fat (g)	22.4	1.5
Saturated Fat (g)	3	0.2
Monounsaturated Fat (g)	6	0.3
Polyunsaturated Fat (g)	12	1
Trans Fatty Acid (g)	0	0
Cholesterol (g)	0	0
Omega-6 Linoleic (g)	0.16	0.17
Omega-3 Linolenic (g)	0.27	0.58
Fiber (g)	4.3	4.7
Sugar (g)	6	7.3
Water (L)	0.24	0.4
Thiamin (mg)	0.2	0.2
Riboflavin (mg)	0.1	0.1
Niacin (mg)	2	1.6
Vitamin B6 (mg)	0.56	0.4
Vitamin B12 (mcg)	0	0
Folate (DFE) mcg	36	40.5
Vitamin C (mg)	25	23.9
Vitamin D (mcg)	0	0
Vitamin A (RAE) (mcg)	199	229.4
Vitamin E (mg)	3.6	20
Calcium (mg)	42	58.5
Iron (mg)	0.82	1.6
Magnesium (mg)	42	48
Potassium (mg)	720	632
Zinc (mg)	0.6	0.66
Sodium (mg)	13	13.1

Portion 1 Cup

Number of Exchanges

Traditional Recipe
1 starchy vegetable exchange
3/4 non-starchy vegetable exchange
5 fat exchange (PUFA)

Healthy Recipe
2/3 starchy vegetable exchange
1 non-starchy vegetable exchange
1 fat exchange (Omega-3-FA)

Calories from Macronutrients

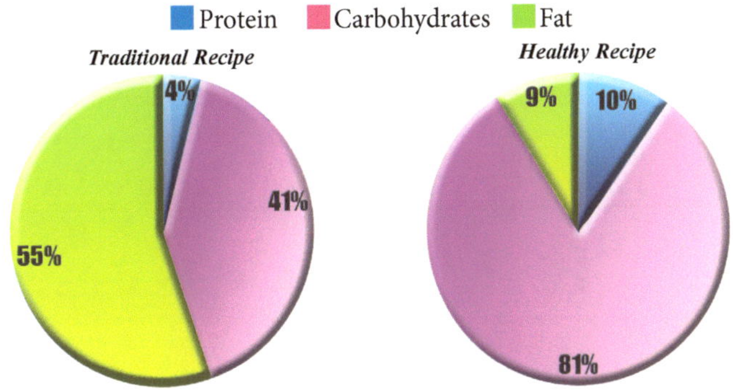

% Fiber Intake Compared to Average Daily Needs

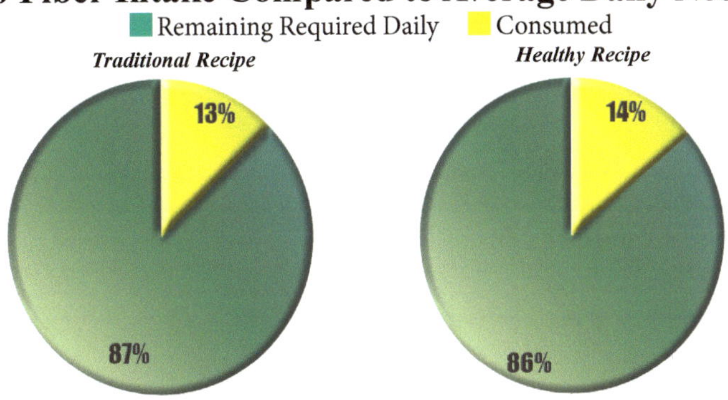

Recommended Portion Sizes & Meal Combinations

Traditional Recipe
(Calorie Controlled)

Men
1 3/4 cups of mahmous
2 slices of small white pita bread

Women
1 cup of mahmous
1 1/2 slices of small white pita bread

Healthy Recipe
(Calorie Controlled & Content Balanced)

Men
3 cups of mahmous
2 slices of small whole wheat pita bread
2 cups of green salad-drizzled with olive oil & vinegar
1 cup of lowfat ayran

Women
1 1/2 cups of mahmous
1 1/2 slices of small whole wheat pita bread
1 1/2 cups of green salad-drizzled with olive oil & vinegar
1 cup of lowfat ayran

Number of Exchanges in a Balanced Meal

Men
2 starchy vegetable exchange
5 non-starchy vegetable exchange
4 fat exchange (3 Omega-3-FA, 1 MUFA)
2 grain exchange
1 milk exchange

Women
1 starchy vegetable exchange
3 non-starchy vegetable exchange
1 3/4 fat exchange (1 Omega-3-FA, 3/4 MUFA)
1 1/2 grain exchange
1 milk exchange

Sautéed Artichoke Topped with Meat

(Angenar Be Al-Lahem)

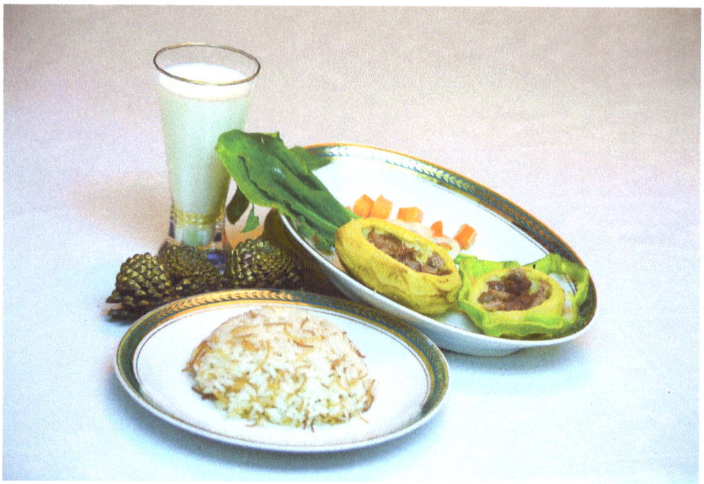

Traditional Recipe, 4 Servings, 4 Cups:

3 1/2 cups or 8 Artichoke Bottoms~520g
6 oz. Ground Medium Fat Meat~168g
7 Tablespoon Corn Oil~96g
2 teaspoons Black Pepper~4g
1/2 cup Lemon Juice~120g
5 cups Water

Traditional Method of Preparation:

- Wash artichoke, drain well
- In a medium pan, add 5 cups of water and add artichoke; boil gently over high heat for 20 minutes
- Season meat with black pepper
- In a saucepan, heat oil and fry meat over medium heat for 10 minutes, until meat is brown
- Add artichoke in cooking pan; top each with cooked meat and add lemon juice
- Cover and cook over medium heat for 5 minutes until juice evaporates
- Ready to serve

Healthy Recipe, 4 Servings, 4 Cups:

3 1/2 cup or 8 Artichoke Bottoms~520g
5.7 oz. Lean Ground Meat~164g
2 teaspoons Corn Oil~9g
2 teaspoons Black Pepper~4g
1/2 cup Lemon Juice~120g
1 cup Water

Healthy Method of Preparation:

- In a steamer, drop 1 tablespoon of lemon juice inside of the artichoke bottoms; turn steamer on to high heat for 30 minutes until artichoke bottoms are tender
- In a non-stick skillet, place ground meat with 4 tablespoons of lemon juice after seasoning with black pepper, and cook over medium heat for 20 minutes until meat is brown
- In a cooking pan, arrange steamed artichoke, top each with cooked meat, add 1 cup of water and 3 tablespoons of lemon juice, and cook over medium heat for anther 7 minutes
- Turn stove off, arrange artichoke in serving plate; brush each artichoke bottom with corn oil
- Ready to serve

Nutritional Goal

Modification of this recipe is essential since fat is the predominant macronutrient in the traditional recipe; fat of the traditional recipe provides more than 70% of total calories. The modification aims to reduce total calories, to improve quality of fat, and to increase nutritional values of food. The calorie content of the healthy recipe is reduced by more than half, when compared to the traditional recipe. The quantity and quality of fat are also controlled; total fat, saturated fat, and cholesterol are reduced by more than 80%, 75% and 10% respectively. A comparison between nutritional analysis of both recipes show that both recipes are nutrient condensed; however, the healthy recipe is enriched with more vitamin B6, niacin, zinc, and potassium, when compared to the traditional recipe. The healthy recipe is recommended to individuals with compromised immune system and excessive body weight.

Nutrient Content	Traditional Recipe	Healthy Recipe
Portion	2 pieces	2 pieces
Weight (g)	381	203.5
Kilocalories (kcal)	370.44	139
Protein (g)	12.55	13.14
Carbohydrate (g)	12.78	11.8
Fat (g)	30.36	4.35
Saturated Fat (g)	5.5	1.22
Monounsaturated Fat (g)	8.58	1.44
Polyunsaturated Fat (g)	14.29	1.44
Trans Fatty Acid (g)	0.46	0.15
Cholesterol (g)	28.55	25.42
Omega-6 Linoleic (g)	14.08	1.4
Omega-3 Linolenic (g)	0.19	0.03
Fiber (g)	2.89	2.57
Sugar (g)	2.45	2.43
Water (L)	0.05	0.06
Thiamin (mg)	0.029	0.02
Riboflavin (mg)	0.072	0.07
Niacin (mg)	2	2.29
Vitamin B6 (mg)	0.168	0.18
Vitamin B12 (mcg)	0.91	0.92
Folate (DFE) mcg	6.48	6.5
Vitamin C (mg)	22.39	23.5
Vitamin D (mcg)	0	0
Vitamin A (RAE) (mcg)	69.51	64.97
Vitamin E (mg)	4.09	0.42
Calcium (mg)	17.7	10.76
Iron (mg)	3.08	2.77
Magnesium (mg)	13.5	13.15
Potassium (mg)	188.56	198.1
Zinc (mg)	1.93	2.12
Sodium (mg)	226.75	213.3

Portion 1 Cup

Number of Exchanges

Traditional Recipe
1 non-starchy vegetable exchange
1 1/3 meat exchange(medium fat)
5 1/3 fat exchange (PUFA)

Healthy Recipe
1 non-starchy vegetable exchange
1 1/3 meat exchange(lean)
1/2 fat exchange (PUFA)

Calories from Macronutrients

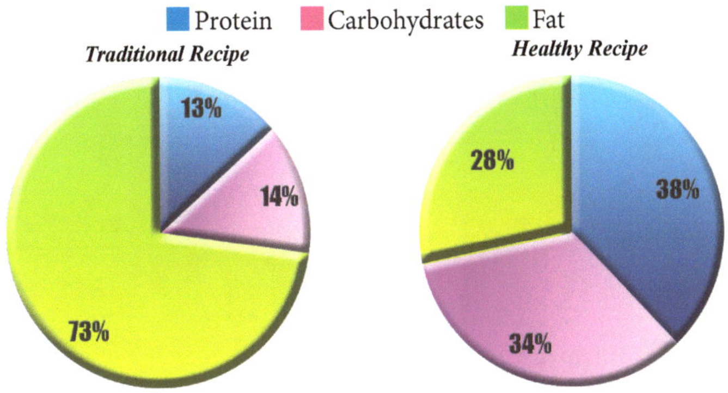

% Fiber Intake Compared to Average Daily Needs

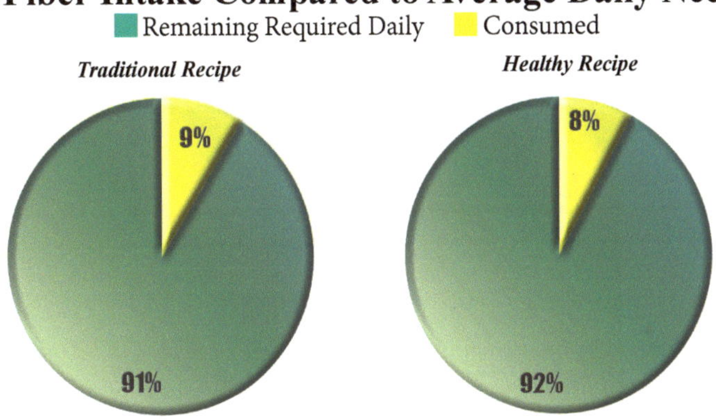

Recommended Portion Sizes & Meal Combinations

Traditional Recipe
(Calorie Controlled)

Men
2 pieces of meat-topped artichoke
3/4 cup of egg noodle rice

Women
1 piece of meat-topped artichoke
1/2 cup of egg noodle rice

Healthy Recipe
(Calorie Controlled & Content Balanced)

Men
4 pieces of meat-topped artichoke
3/4 cup egg noodle rice
(see page:128)
1 cup green salad–drizzled with olive oil
1 cup lowfat ayran

Women
2 pieces of meat-topped artichoke
1/2 cup of egg noodle rice
(see page:128)
3/4 cup green salad-drizzled with olive oil
1 cup lowfat ayran

Number of Exchanges in a Balanced Meal

Men
3 fat exchange (2 PUFA, 1 MUFA)
3 grain exchange
2 2/3 meat exchange (lean)
2 2/3 non-starchy vegetable exchange
1 milk exchange

Women
2 fat exchange (1 1/4PUFA, 3/4 MUFA)
2 grain exchange
1 1/3 meat exchange (lean)
1 3/4 non-starchy vegetable exchange
1 milk exchange

115

Sautéed Artichoke Topped with Vegetables

(Angenar Be Al-Khodar)

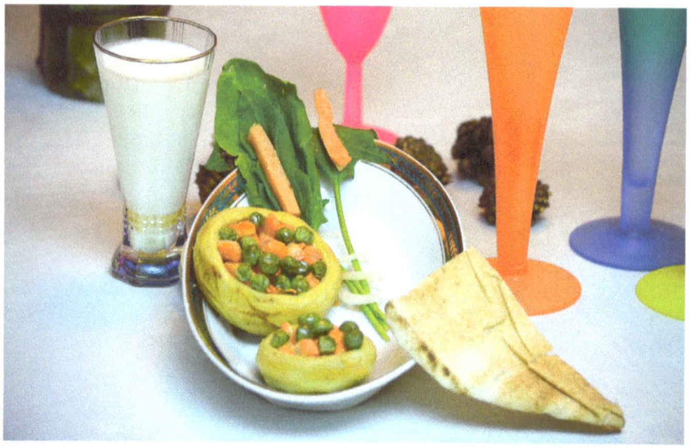

Traditional Recipe, 4 Servings, 4 Cups:

1 cup Shredded Onion~160g
3 1/4 cups or 8 bottoms Artichoke~482g
1/2 cup Diced Carrots~80g
1/3 cup Fresh Green Peas~60g
1/2 cup Fresh Lemon Juice~120g
2 1/2 Tablespoons Olive Oil~36g
7 Tablespoons Corn Oil~96g
1 Tablespoon of Lemon Salt (Optional)
10 cups Water

Traditional Method of Preparation:

- Wash artichoke, drain well
- In a medium pan, dissolve lemon salt in 8 cups of water and add artichokes. Boil gently over high heat for 20 minutes
- In a saucepan, heat oil and fry onions over medium heat for 5 minutes
- In a cooking pan, combine olive oil, peas and carrots and cook on medium heat for 10 minutes until vegetables are tender
- Reduce heat, combine onion, carrots and peas with 2 cups of water, cook over low heat for 10 minutes, until water evaporates
- Add lemon juice to vegetables and stir for 2 minutes
- In a serving plate arrange artichoke bottoms top each with 1/4 cup of vegetables
- Ready to serve

Healthy Recipe, 4 Servings, 4 Cups:

1 cup Shredded Onion~161g
3 1/4 cups or 8 bottoms Artichoke~482g
1 cup Diced Carrots~159g
1/3 cup Fresh Green Peas~62g
1/4 cup Lemon Juice~60g
4 1/2 teaspoons Olive Oil~21g
1 teaspoon Ground Flaxseed~2.5g
1 cup Water

Healthy Method of Preparation:

- Steam carrots, peas and artichokes separately
  Pour 1 tablespoon of lemon juice into the artichoke bottom: turn steamer on to high heat for 30 minutes until vegetables are tender
- In a saucepan, place onions with 1 cup of water and cook over high heat for 15 minutes, until the onions are juicy and the water evaporates
- Combine steamed carrots and peas with onions; add 3 tablespoons of lemon juice and cook for another 5 minutes
- Turn stove off; add flaxseed and 3 teaspoons of olive oil to vegetables and cover tightly
- In serving plate arrange artichoke bottoms, brush each artichoke bottom with olive oil and top it with 1/4 cup of vegetables
- Ready to serve

Nutritional Goal

The modification of this recipe is essential since fat is the predominant in the traditional recipe, calories from fat are 70% of total calories. The calorie content of the healthy recipe is reduced by more than half when compared to the calorie content of the traditional recipe. Calories from macronutrients are balanced after more than 80% reduction in total fat. Quality of fat is improved since saturated fat is reduced by more than 75%. The healthy cooking method preserves the quality of oil and avoids the transition of healthy fat into bad fat. The nutritional analysis comparison between two recipes shows that the healthy recipe contains more than 4% fiber, 10% thiamin, 30% niacin, 20% calcium, 20% magnesium, and 15% more potassium. The healthy recipe is recommended to individuals with anemia, osteoporosis, digestive problems, high lipid profiles, and excessive body weight.

Nutrient Content	Traditional Recipe	Healthy Recipe
Portion	2 pieces	2 pieces
Weight (g)	353	229
Kilocalories (kcal)	387	139.28
Protein (g)	5.3	5.11
Carbohydrate (g)	19	17.43
Fat (g)	33	5.78
Saturated Fat (g)	4.28	0.77
Monounsaturated Fat (g)	12.47	4.03
Polyunsaturated Fat (g)	15	0.78
Trans Fatty Acid (g)	0.68	0
Cholesterol (g)	0	0
Omega-6 Linoleic (g)	14.77	0.53
Omega-3 Linolenic (g)	0.244	0.19
Fiber (g)	4.17	4.4
Sugar (g)	6	7
Water (L)	0.09	0.14
Thiamin (mg)	0.07	0.08
Riboflavin (mg)	0.04	0.04
Niacin (mg)	0.48	0.629
Vitamin B6 (mg)	0.13	0.131
Vitamin B12 (mcg)	0	0
Folate (DFE) mcg	28.75	25.4
Vitamin C (mg)	27.8	21.23
Vitamin D (mcg)	0	0
Vitamin A (RAE) (mcg)	933	1750
Vitamin E (mg)	5.13	0.63
Calcium (mg)	22.79	27.67
Iron (mg)	1.97	1.97
Magnesium (mg)	14.3	17.4
Potassium (mg)	192	223.4
Zinc (mg)	0.3	0.36
Sodium	193.8	185.8

Portion 1 Cup

Number of Exchanges

Traditional Recipe
1 non-starchy vegetable exchange
7 1/43 fat exchange
(5 1/4 PUFA, 2 MUFA)

Healthy Recipe
1 1/3 non-starchy vegetable exchange
1 1/4 fat exchange
(1MUFA, 1/4 Omega-3-FA)

Calories from Macronutrients

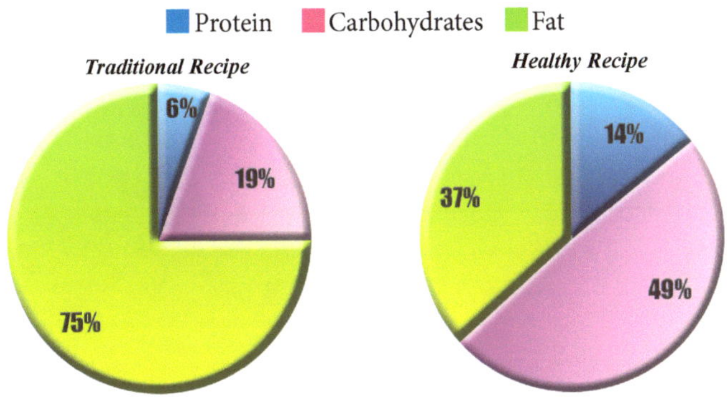

% Fiber Intake Compared to Average Daily Needs

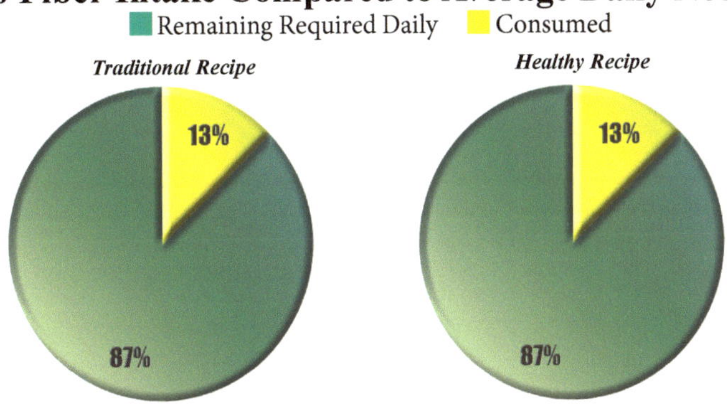

Recommended Portion Sizes & Meal Combinations

Traditional Recipe
(Calorie Controlled)

Men
3 1/2 pieces of angenar be al-khodar
1 1/2 slices of small white pita bread

Women
2 pieces of angenar be al-khodar
1 slices of small white pita bread

Healthy Recipe
(Calorie Controlled & Content Balanced)

Men
7 pieces of angenar be al-khodar
3 slices of small whole wheat pita bread
1 cup low fat ayran

Women
4 pieces of angenar be al-khodar
2 slices of small whole wheat pita bread
1 cup low fat ayran

Number of Exchanges in a Balanced Meal

Men
4 1/2 non-starchy vegetable exchange
5 fat exchange (4 MUFA,
1 Omega-3-FA)
3 grain exchange
1 milk exchange
1/2 meat exchange (very lean)
1/2 starch exchange

Women
2 2/3 non-starchy vegetable exchange
2 3/4 fat exchange (2 1/4 MUFA,
1/2 Omega-3-FA)
2 grain exchange
1 milk exchange
1/3 meat exchange (very lean)
1/3 starch exchange

Spinach Stewed with Ground Meat

(Sabanekh Be Al-Lahem)

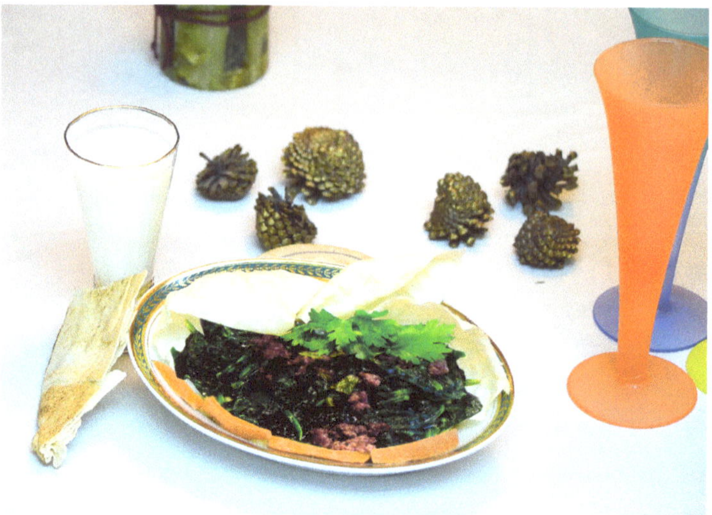

Traditional Recipe, 4 Servings, 4 Cups:

10 1/4 cups Fresh Chopped Spinach~806.4g
1 1/4 cups Chopped Onions~192g
30 oz. Ground Meat~371.2g
1 2/3 cups Fresh Lemon Juice~390.4g
2 3/4 Tablespoons Fresh Chopped Cilantro~35.2g
3/4 cup Corn Oil~172.8g
1 cup Water

Traditional Method of Preparation:

- Season meat with black pepper
- In a skillet, heat oil and fry onions over medium heat for 3 minutes
- Combine meat with onions, continue frying and stirring for 5 minutes, until meat is brown
- Add spinach and 1 cup of water to onions and meat
- Cover and cook over medium heat for 10 minutes
- Add cilantro and lemon juice; stir twice
- Turn stove off; set for 5 minutes
- Ready to serve

Healthy Recipe, 4 Servings, 4 Cups:

5 cups Fresh Chopped Spinach~399.56g
10 Tablespoons Chopped Onions~101.16g
5.3 oz. Lean Ground Meat~151.6g
10 Tablespoons Fresh Lemon Juice~101.16g
2 3/4 Tablespoons Fresh Chopped Cilantro~35.2g
3/4 Tablespoon Corn Oil~10.8g
1 2/3 teaspoons Ground Flaxseed~12.64g
2 1/4 cups Water

Healthy Method of Preparation:

- Steam spinach at high heat for 20 minutes
- Season meat with black pepper, and place in a skillet with 3/4 cup of water over medium heat for 10 minutes. Drain and store meat broth in refrigerator
- Bring onion and 1/2 cup of water to boil for 5 minutes, until onions are thick and juicy
- Combine 1 cup of water with spinach, meat and onions; cover and cook over medium heat for 15 minutes, until water evaporates
- Reduce heat, add lemon juice and cilantro, and cook over low heat for 3 minutes; stir constantly to prevent sticking
- Turn stove off, add corn oil
- Ready to serve

Nutritional Goal

The modification of traditional recipe is essential since fat is the predominant macronutrient. More than 70% of total calories is from fat. The healthy method of preparation preserves the quality of fat and conserves the volume of food. In the healthy recipe, total fat, saturated fat, and trans fatty acid are reduced by more than 80%, and cholesterol is reduced by more than 60%, when compared to the traditional recipe. Also, the calories content of the healthy recipe is reduced by more than 70%, and the ratio of omega-6: omega-3 promotes heart health. Although the healthy recipe has less nutrient contents than the traditional recipe, the macronutrient contents of the healthy recipe are more balanced, and the high caloric of traditional recipe compensates its nutrient contents. Following the recommended portion sizes and meal combinations provides an adequate nutritional value for individuals.

Nutrient Content	Traditional Recipe	Healthy Recipe
Portion	1 cup	1 cup
Weight (g)	240	234
Kilocalories (kcal)	679.6	125.4
Protein (g)	24.3	11.9
Carbohydrate (g)	21.46	7.1
Fat (g)	58	6.5
Saturated Fat (g)	11	1.4
Monounsaturated Fat (g)	17	1.8
Polyunsaturated Fat (g)	26	2.9
Trans Fatty Acid (g)	0.99	0.14
Cholesterol (g)	63	23.5
Omega-6 Linoleic (g)	25.6	1.8
Omega-3 Linolenic (g)	0.6	0.89
Fiber (g)	5.9	3.35
Sugar (g)	5.6	1.3
Water (L)	0.39	0.4
Thiamin (mg)	0.28	0.17
Riboflavin (mg)	0.5	0.27
Niacin (mg)	6	3
Vitamin B6 (mg)	0.8	0.38
Vitamin B12 (mcg)	2	0.85
Folate (DFE) mcg	430	206.43
Vitamin C (mg)	105.9	40.39
Vitamin D (mcg)	0	0
Vitamin A (RAE) (mcg)	5785	2860.5
Vitamin E (mg)	10.9	2.15
Calcium (mg)	236.3	114.3
Iron (mg)	8	3.98
Magnesium (mg)	189.7	102.4
Potassium (mg)	1634	764.2
Zinc (mg)	5.5	2.66
Sodium (mg)	223.4	105.4

Portion 1 Cup

Number of Exchanges

Traditional Recipe
3 non-starchy vegetable exchange
3 meat exchange (medium fat)
9 2/3 fat exchange (PUFA)

Healthy Recipe
1 1/3 non-starchy vegetable exchange
1 1/4 meat exchange (lean)
1 fat exchange (1/3 Omega-3-FA, 2/3 PUFA)

Calories from Macronutrients

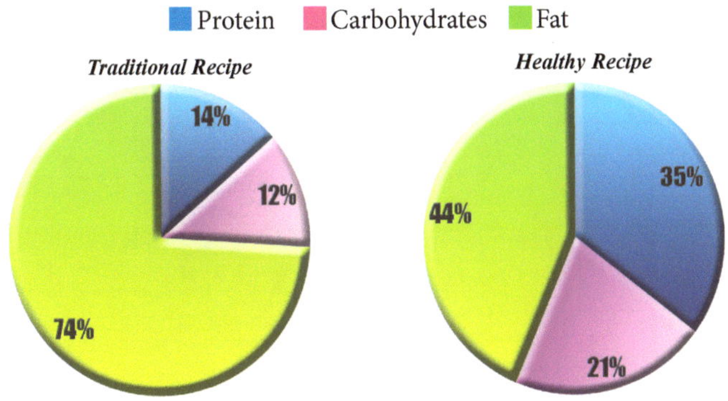

% Fiber Intake Compared to Average Daily Needs

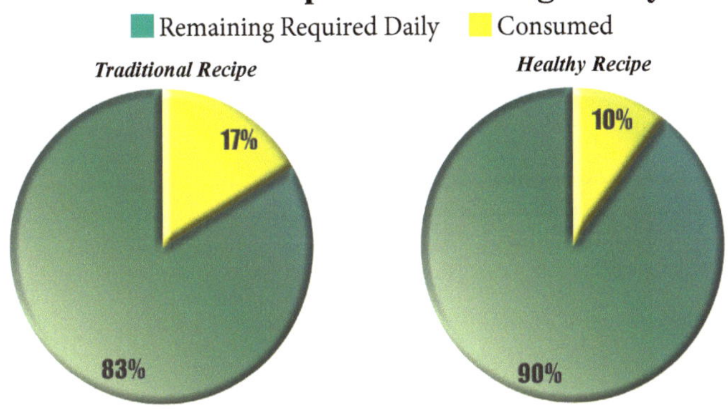

Recommended Portion Sizes & Meal Combinations

Traditional Recipe
(Calorie Controlled)

Men
1 cup of sabanekh be al-lahem
1 1/2 slices of small white pita bread

Women
2/3 cup of sabanekh be al-lahem
1/2 slice of small white pita bread

Healthy Recipe
(Calorie Controlled & Content Balanced)

Men
4 cups of sabanekh be al-lahem
3 slices of small whole wheat pita bread
1 cup of lowfat ayran

Women
2 1/2 cups of sabanekh be al-lahem
1 1/2 slice of small whole wheat pita bread
1 cup of lowfat ayran

Number of Exchanges in a Balanced Meal

Men
1 milk exchange
3 grain exchange
5 2/3 non-starchy vegetable exchange
2 fat exchange (1 2/3 Omega-3-FA,2 1/4 PUFA)
5 meat exchange (lean)

Women
1 milk exchange
1 1/2 grain exchange
3 1/2 non-starchy vegetable exchange
2 1/3 fat exchange (1 Omega-3-FA,1 1/3 PUFA)
3 meat exchange (lean)

Spinach Sautéed with Olive Oil & Cilantro

(Sabanekh Be Al-Zayet)

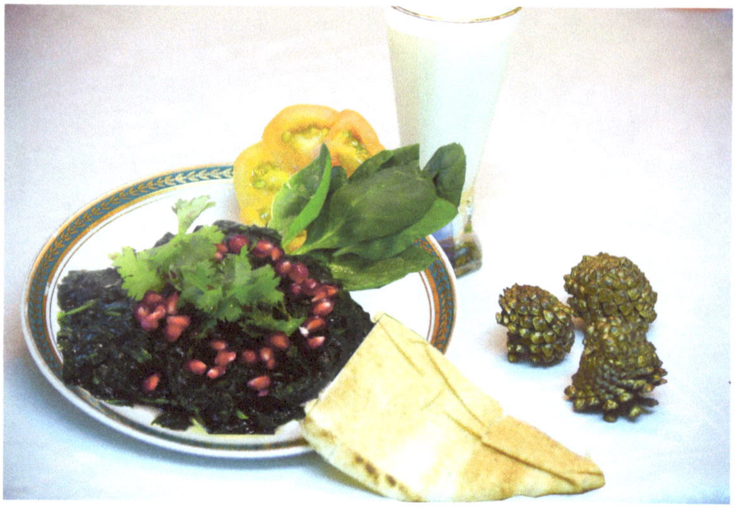

Traditional Recipe, 4 Servings, 4 Cups:

- 10 cups Fresh Chopped Spinach~792.6g
- 1 1/2 cups Chopped Onions~229.6g
- 15 Tablespoons Olive Oil~200g
- 3 3/4 Tablespoons Ground Garlic~44.4g
- 3 1/2 Tablespoons Fresh Chopped Cilantro~44.4g
- 5 cups Water

Traditional Method of Preparation:

- Wash and drain spinach
- In a cooking pan, heat olive oil and fry onions over medium heat for 5 minutes
- Combine spinach with onions, continue frying for 5 minutes
- Add 5 cups of water; cook over medium heat for 15 minutes, until water evaporates
- Add cilantro and garlic, stir continuously for 3 minutes
- Ready to serve

Healthy Recipe, 4 Servings, 4 Cups:

- 8 1/2 cups Fresh Chopped Spinach~672g
- 1 cup Chopped Onions~160g
- 2 2/3 Tablespoons Olive Oil~36g
- 4 teaspoons Ground Garlic~16g
- 5 Tablespoons Fresh Chopped Cilantro~64g
- 1 cup Water

Healthy Method of Preparation:

- Steam spinach at high heat for 15 minutes
- Combine chopped cilantro and garlic with spinach; steam for 5 minutes
- In a cooking pan, combine 1 cup of water with onions; bring it to a gentle boil for 8 minutes, until onions are thick and juicy
- Add steamed spinach with cilantro, garlic and onions. Stir twice over medium heat for 1 minute
- Place the food on a serving plate; drizzled with olive oil while food is hot
- Ready to serve

Nutritional Goal

The purpose of modification is to save calories, to balance macronutrients proportion, and to preserve the quality of fat. The modification of this recipe is essential since more than 80% of total calories are fat calories. The total calories of the healthy recipe are reduced by more than 70% when compared to the total calories of the traditional recipe. Changing the cooking method preserves the quality of fat and prevents the transition of fat into bad fat during cooking. Although the traditional recipe has more nutrient contents than healthy recipe, the difference in nutrient values is insignificant when compared to the difference in quality and quantity of fat in both recipes. The healthy recipe is recommended to individuals seeking healthier lifestyles.

Nutrient Content	Traditional Recipe	Healthy Recipe
Portion	1 cup	1 cup
Weight (g)	248.168	232
Kilocalories (kcal)	530.5	143.44
Protein (g)	7.15	5.77
Carbohydrate (g)	17	12.1
Fat (g)	50.9	9.6
Saturated Fat (g)	6.88	1.33
Monounsaturated Fat (g)	36.9	6.6
Polyunsaturated Fat (g)	5.4	1.2
Trans Fatty Acid (g)	0	0
Cholesterol (g)	0	0
Omega-6 Linoleic (g)	4.69	0.88
Omega-3 Linolenic (g)	0.67	0.3
Fiber (g)	5.6	4.7
Sugar (g)	3.6	2.7
Water (L)	0.25	0.2
Thiamin (mg)	0.22	0.18
Riboflavin (mg)	0.4	0.35
Niacin (mg)	1.67	1.4
Vitamin B6 (mg)	0.6	0.45
Vitamin B12 (mcg)	0	0
Folate (DFE) mcg	401.5	341.8
Vitamin C (mg)	63.4	51.89
Vitamin D (mcg)	0	0
Vitamin A (RAE) (mcg)	5656.1	4809.6
Vitamin E (mg)	8.3	3.78
Calcium (mg)	232.1	186.2
Iron (mg)	6.2	5.1
Magnesium (mg)	166.6	139.9
Potassium (mg)	1255.9	1042.9
Zinc (mg)	1.33	1.1
Sodium (mg)	161.8	135

Portion 1 Cup

Number of Exchanges

Traditional Recipe
3 non-starchy vegetable exchange
11 fat exchange (MUFA)

Healthy Recipe
2 1/2 non-starchy vegetable exchange
2 fat exchange (MUFA)

Calories from Macronutrients

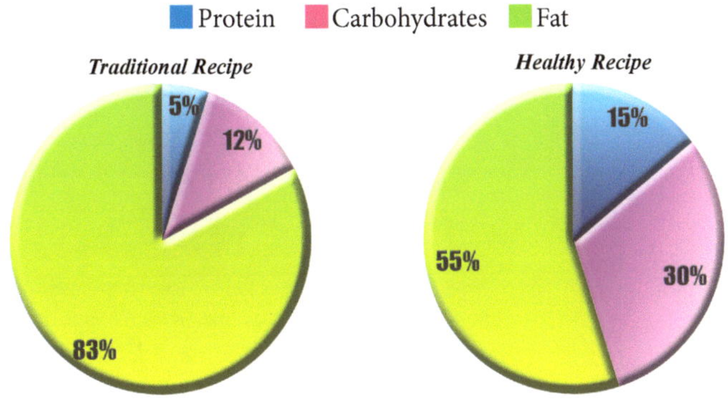

% Fiber Intake Compared to Average Daily Needs

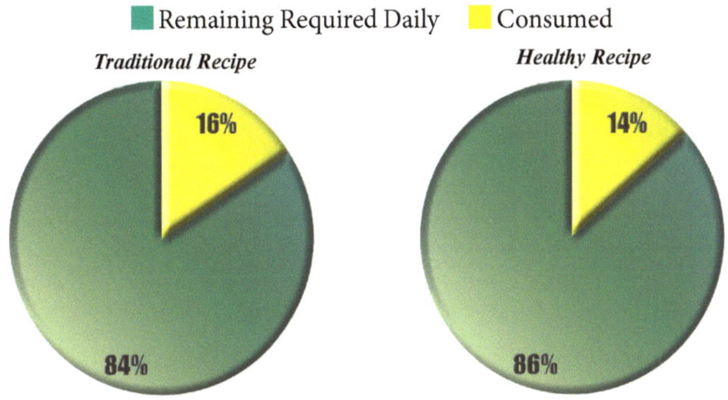

Recommended Portion Sizes & Meal Combinations

Traditional Recipe
(Calorie Controlled)

Men
1 1/4 cups of sabanekh be al-zayet
1 1/2 slices of small white pita bread

Women
3/4 cup of sabanekh be al-zayet
1 slice of small white pita bread

Healthy Recipe
(Calorie Controlled & Content Balanced)

Men
3 1/2 cups of sabanekh be al-zayet
2 1/2 slices of small whole wheat pita bread
1 cup of lowfat ayran

Women
2 cups of sabanekh be al-zayet
1 1/2 slices of small whole wheat pita bread
1 cup of lowfat ayran

Number of Exchanges in a Balanced Meal

Men
1 milk exchange
2 1/2 grain exchange
8 2/3 non-starchy vegetable exchange
6 2/3 fat exchange (MUFA)

Women
1 milk exchange
1 1/2 grain exchange
5 non-starchy vegetable exchange
4 fat exchange (MUFA)

Tomatoes Stewed with Meat & Cilantro

(Monazal Al-Ahmar)

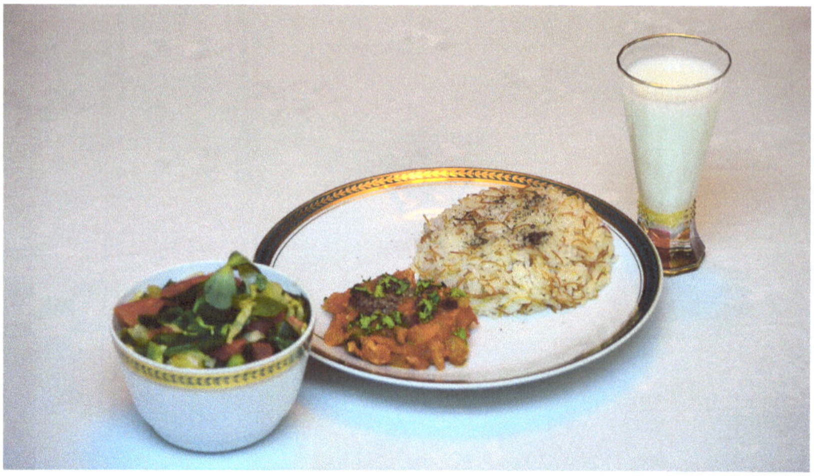

Traditional Recipe, 4 Servings, 4 Cups:

6 oz. Medium Fat Ground Meat~172.7g
2 1/3 Tablespoons Fresh Chopped Cilantro~30.3g
5 1/2 cups Peeled Diced Tomatoes~1327g
1 1/2 teaspoons Ground Garlic~6g
2 teaspoons Black Pepper~4g
2 Tablespoons Corn Oil~27.27g

Traditional Method of Preparation:

- Wash tomatoes carefully; soak in warm water for 3 minutes until they are easy to peel
- Cut peeled tomatoes into quarters
- Season meat with black pepper
- Heat oil and fry meat over medium heat for 5 minutes until meat is brown
- Add tomatoes and stir twice, cover and cook for 30 minutes
- Add cilantro and garlic; stir twice
- Reduce heat; continue cooking over low heat for another 3 minutes
- Ready to serve

Healthy Recipe, 4 Servings, 4 Cups:

3.6 oz. Lean Meat~103.5g
5 1/2 Tablespoon Fresh Chopped Cilantro~72.4g
3 cups Diced Tomatoes~766.1g
1 1/2 Tablespoon Ground Garlic~20.7g
2 teaspoons Black Pepper~4g
1 2/3 Tablespoons Tomato Paste~26.9g
1 2/3 Tablespoons Ground Flaxseed~12.9g
4 cups Water

Healthy Method of Preparation:

- Cut tomatoes into quarters
- Season meat with black pepper
- In a deep cooking pan, place meat with tomato paste and 4 cups of water; cook over medium heat for 10 minutes until meat is reddish-brown
- Add tomatoes to pan, cover and cook over medium heat for 30 minutes
- Add cilantro and garlic; stir twice
- Turn stove off, sprinkle flaxseed and stir twice
- Simmer for 3 minutes
- Ready to serve

  Optional: Keep broiled meat aside to garnish cooked tomatoes

Nutritional Goal

The purpose of modification is to reduce calories content, to balance calories from macronutrients, and to improve omega-6: omega-3 ratio. Calories of the healthy recipe are reduced by more than half when compared to calories of the traditional recipe. Fat control and healthy method of preparation balance the calories from macronutrients. In the healthy recipe total fat, saturated fat, and trans fatty acid are reduced by more than 70%, cholesterol is also reduced by half comparing to their levels in the traditional recipe. The addition of flaxseed improves the ratio of omega-3: omega-6 in the healthy recipe, which promotes the health of the heart. The omitting of corn oil saves volume of tomato when cooking; therefore, less tomato is added resulting in reduction in fiber content. Nevertheless, following the recommended portion sizes and meal content is encouraged to increase the fiber intake in this meal. The healthy recipe is recommended to individuals with high lipid profiles and excessive body weight.

Nutrient Content	Traditional Recipe	Healthy Recipe
Portion	1 cup	1 cup
Weight (g)	221.96	263.99
Kilocalories (kcal)	276.414	106.5
Protein (g)	9.8	8.8
Carbohydrate (g)	16	12
Fat (g)	21	3.1
Saturated Fat (g)	6	0.8
Monounsaturated Fat (g)	7.5	0.9
Polyunsaturated Fat (g)	4.8	1.3
Trans Fatty Acid (g)	0.81	0.1
Cholesterol (g)	34	16
Omega-6 Linoleic (g)	4.7	0.33
Omega-3 Linolenic (g)	0.1	0.75
Fiber (g)	4.4	4
Sugar (g)	8.9	6.4
Water (L)	0.35	0.45
Thiamin (mg)	0.17	0.17
Riboflavin (mg)	0.14	0.12
Niacin (mg)	3.6	3.1
Vitamin B6 (mg)	0.5	0.4
Vitamin B12 (mcg)	0.9	0.6
Folate (DFE) mcg	57	43.2
Vitamin C (mg)	45	28.4
Vitamin D (mcg)	0	0
Vitamin A (RAE) (mcg)	855	556
Vitamin E (mg)	2.3	1.1
Calcium (mg)	59.9	45.78
Iron (mg)	2	2
Magnesium (mg)	47	46
Potassium (mg)	930	695
Zinc (mg)	2.2	2
Sodium (mg)	47	82

Portion 1 Cup

Number of Exchanges

Traditional Recipe	Healthy Recipe
1 1/3 meat exchange (medium fat)	1 meat exchange (lean)
1 1/3 non-starchy vegetable exchange	1 non-starchy vegetable exchange
1 1/2 fat exchange (PUFA)	1 1/4 fat exchange (Omega-3-FA)

Calories from Macronutrients

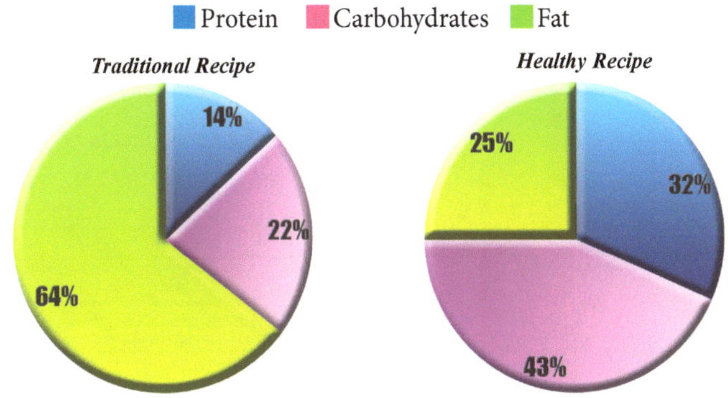

% Fiber Intake Compared to Average Daily Needs

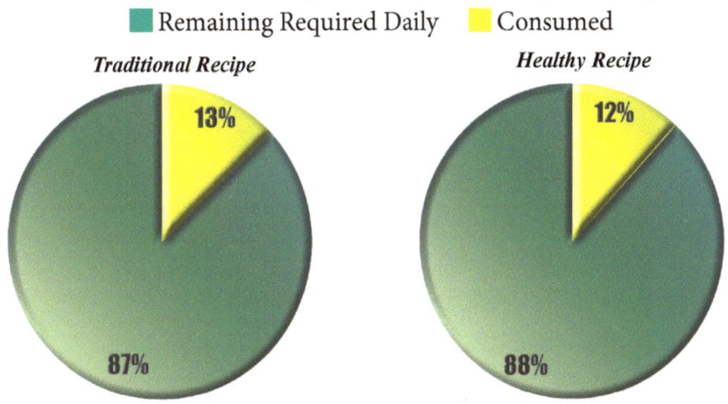

Recommended Portion Sizes & Meal Combinations

Traditional Recipe
(Calorie Controlled)

Ment
1 1/2 cups of monazal al-ahmar
2/3 cup of traditional egg noodle rice

Women
3/4 cup of monazal al-ahmar
1/2 cup of traditional egg noodle rice

Healthy Recipe
(Calorie Controlled & Content Balanced)

Men
3 cups of monazal al-ahmar
3/4 cup of healthy egg noodle rice (see page:128)
2 cups of green salad-drizzled with vinegar
1 cup of lowfat ayran

Women
1 1/2 cups of monazal al-ahmar
1/2 cups of healthy egg noodle rice (see page:!28)
1 1/2 cups of green salad-drizzled with vinegar
1 cup of lowfat ayran

Number of Exchanges in a Balanced Meal

Men
4 2/3 non-starchy vegetable exchange
2 1/3 meat exchange (lean)
3 grain exchange
1 milk exchange
4 2/3 fat exchange (3 2/3 Omega-3-FA, 1 PUFA)

Women
3 non-starchy vegetable exchange
1 1/4 meat exchange (lean)
2 grain exchange
1 milk exchange
2 3/4 fat exchange
(3/4 PUFA, 2 Omega-3-FA)

Vegetables with Meat Stewed in Tomato Base

(Kawag)

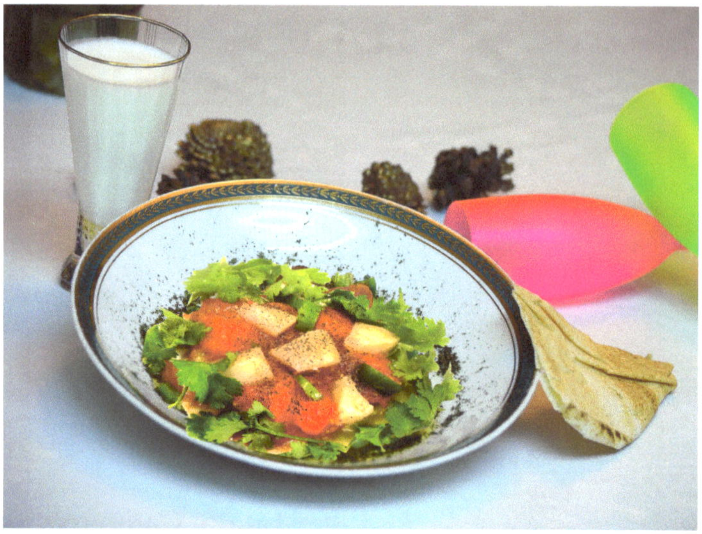

Traditional Recipe, 4 Servings, 4 Cups:

1/2 cup Shredded Onions~78g
1 1/3 cups Chopped Green Pepper~171.24g
2 2/3 cups Diced Tomatoes~630g
1 3/4 cups Diced Potatoes~ 408g
1 1/4 cups Diced Zucchini~240g
3 oz. Shank Meat~84g
8 cups water

Traditional Method of Preparation:

- Broil meat with 8 cups of water over medium-high heat for 15 minutes
- Combine all ingredients with meat, cover and cook over low-medium heat for 40 minutes
- Turn stove off; leave for 5 minutes
- Ready to serve

Healthy Recipe, 4 Servings, 4 Cups:

1/3 cup Shredded Onions~52g
1 cup Chopped Green Pepper~114.4g
1 3/4 cups Diced Tomatoes~421.2g
3/4 cup Diced Potato~176.8g
3/4 cup Diced Zucchini~161.2g
2 oz. Lean Shank meat~54g
5 1/4 teaspoons Ground Flaxseed~13g
6 Tablespoons Ground Oatmeal~36g
9 cups water

Healthy Method of Preparation:

- Broil meat with 9 cups of water over medium-high heat for 15 minutes
- Combine all ingredients with meat, cover and cook over low-medium heat for 40 minutes
- Turn stove off; sprinkle flaxseed and leave for 5 minutes
- Ready to serve

Nutritional Goal

The traditional recipe is considered a healthy food. However, the modification aims to increase fiber and to balance omega-6: omega-3 ratio. The addition of ground oatmeal leads to an increase in fiber of more than 8% in the healthy recipe. The addition of ground flaxseed and the selection of lean meat are reasons for the improvement of omega-6: omega-3 ratio, when compared to the traditional recipe. These valuable changes make the healthy recipe a good choice to individuals with digestive problems and individuals who are at high risk of heart disease.

Nutrient Content	Traditional Recipe	Healthy Recipe
Portion	1 cup	1 cup
Weight (g)	254	254
Kilocalories (kcal)	137.466	135.5
Protein (g)	9.9	8
Carbohydrate (g)	22	22.4
Fat (g)	2.3	2.6
Saturated Fat (g)	0.2	0.44
Monounsaturated Fat (g)	0.1	0.6
Polyunsaturated Fat (g)	0.35	1.3
Trans Fatty Acid (g)	0	0
Cholesterol (g)	0.72	5.3
Omega-6 Linoleic (g)	0.27	0.17
Omega-3 Linolenic (g)	0.08	0.79
Fiber (g)	4.7	5.13
Sugar (g)	8.4	5.8
Water (L)	14.5	11.4
Thiamin (mg)	0.19	0.2
Riboflavin (mg)	0.13	0.1
Niacin (mg)	3.46	2.8
Vitamin B6 (mg)	0.5	0.4
Vitamin B12 (mcg)	0.65	0.45
Folate (DFE) mcg	43.6	35.5
Vitamin C (mg)	87.45	58.6
Vitamin D (mcg)	0	0
Vitamin A (RAE) (mcg)	443.9	297.57
Vitamin E (mg)	0.76	0.57
Calcium (mg)	46.66	42.6
Iron (mg)	2.1	1.85
Magnesium (mg)	59.44	63.2
Potassium (mg)	1140.6	830.6
Zinc (mg)	2.37	2.1
Sodium (mg)	25.8	18.8

Portion 1 Cup

Number of Exchanges

Traditional Recipe
1 1/3 non-starchy vegetable exchange
1 starchy vegetable exchange
2/3 meat exchange (high fat)

Healthy Recipe
1 non-starchy vegetable exchange
1/3 starchy vegetable exchange
1/3 meat exchange (medium fat)
1 1/3 fat exchange (Omega-3-FA)
1/2 grain exchange

Calories from Macronutrients

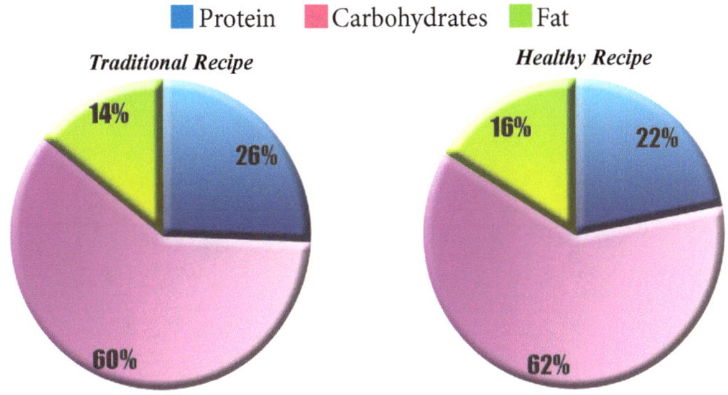

% Fiber Intake Compared to Average Daily Needs

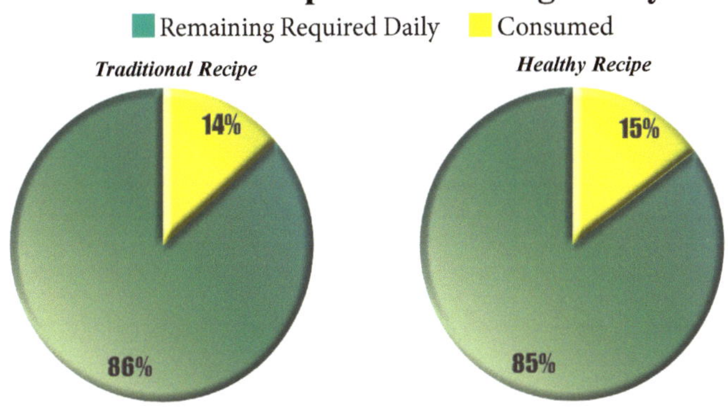

Recommended Portion Sizes & Meal Combinations

Traditional Recipe
(Calorie Controlled)

Men
3 1/2 cups of kawag
3 slices of small white pita bread
1 cup of regular ayran

Women
2 cups of kawag
2 slices of small white pita bread
1 cup of regular ayran

Healthy Recipe
(Calorie Controlled & Content Balanced)

Men
3 1/2 cups of kawag
3 slices of small whole wheat pita bread
1 cup of lowfat ayran

Women
2 cups of kawag
2 slices of small whole wheat pita bread
1 cup of lowfat ayran

Number of Exchanges in a Balanced Meal

Men
3 1/3 non-starchy vegetable exchange
1 1/3 starchy vegetable exchange
4 1/2 fat exchange (Omega-3-FA)
4 3/4 grain exchange
1 1/3 meat exchange (lean)
1 milk exchange

Women
2 non-starchy vegetable exchange
3/4 starchy vegetable exchange
2 2/3 fat exchange (Omega-3-FA)
3 grain exchange
1 meat exchange (lean)
1 milk exchange

Zucchini Stewed with Meat, Chickpeas & Vegetables

(Mosakaa Kousa & Hummus)

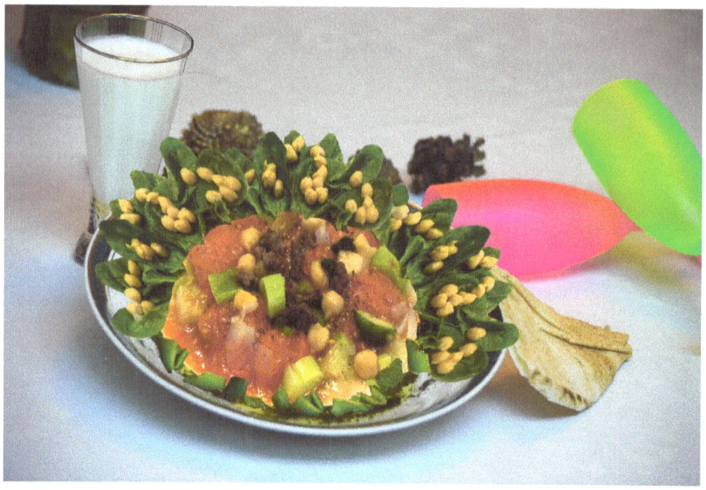

Traditional Recipe, 4 Servings, 4 Cups:

1 2/3 cups Chopped Zucchini~302.8g
1/2 cup Chopped Tomatoes~112g
2/3 cup Soaked Chickpeas~112g
1/2 cup Chopped Onions~65g
4.8 oz. Meat Shank~138g
3 1/2 Tablespoons Corn Oil~46.6g
1 teaspoon Black Pepper~2g
8 cups Water

Healthy Recipe, 4 Servings, 4 Cups:

2 1/3 cups Chopped Zucchini~450.5g
2/3 cup Chopped Tomatoes~157.7g
2/3 cup Soaked Chickpeas~112.5g
1/2 cup Chopped Onions~73g
1.2 oz. Lean Meat Shank~34g
2/3 cup Tomato Juice~140.8g
1/4 teaspoon Black Pepper~ 0.5g
7 cups Water

Traditional Method of Preparation:

- Soak chickpeas over night for 12 hours
- In a cooking pan, heat oil and fry onion over medium heat for 5 minutes; until onions are gold
- Season meat with black pepper and combine with onions; continue to cook over medium heat for 10 minutes; stir frequently to prevent sticking
- Add zucchini and tomatoes; stir twice
- Combine all ingredients together with 8 cups of water and cook over medium heat for 30 minutes until meat and chickpeas are tender
- Ready to serve

Healthy Method of Preparation:

- Soak chickpeas over night for 12 hours
- In a cooking pan, bring 7 cups of water to boil; season meat with black pepper and cook over medium heat for 5 minutes
- Add chickpeas with meat and continue to cook for 10 minutes
- Combine all ingredients together and cook over medium heat for another 10 minutes
- Ready to serve

Nutritional Goal

The purpose of the modification is to reduce calorie content, improve fat quality, improve omega-6: omega-3 ratio, and to enrich food with fiber and nutrients. Calorie content of the healthy recipe is reduced by more than 35% when compared to calorie content of the traditional recipe. Total fat, saturated fat, and cholesterol are greatly reduced by more than 75%, when compared to their levels in the traditional recipe. Thus, fat is no longer the predominant macronutrient in the healthy recipe. A comparison between nutritional analysis of the traditional and the healthy recipes demonstrates that the healthy recipe has greater levels of different nutrients. Fiber content is increased by more than 8%; vitamin C and vitamin A are increased by half. Folate, calcium, iron, potassium and magnesium are increased by more than 5%. The healthy recipe is recommended to individuals with high lipid profiles, excessive body weight, osteoporosis, post menopause, and malnutrition.

Nutrient Content	Traditional Recipe	Healthy Recipe
Portion	1 cup	1 cup
Weight (g)	226	252
Kilocalories (kcal)	270	155.2
Protein (g)	14.5	10.7
Carbohydrate (g)	22.1	25.5
Fat (g)	14.7	2.5
Saturated Fat (g)	2	0.4
Monounsaturated Fat (g)	3.6	0.6
Polyunsaturated Fat (g)	7.6	0.8
Trans Fatty Acid (g)	0.03	0
Cholesterol (g)	25.8	2.6
Omega-6 Linoleic (g)	6.9	0.12
Omega-3 Linolenic (g)	0.2	0.15
Fiber (g)	6.3	7
Sugar (g)	6	8.5
Water (L)	3.4	41
Thiamin (mg)	0.2	0.2
Riboflavin (mg)	0.2	0.14
Niacin (mg)	3.8	2.1
Vitamin B6 (mg)	0.5	0.44
Vitamin B12 (mcg)	0.5	0.3
Folate (DFE) mcg	183.3	196
Vitamin C (mg)	31.5	52
Vitamin D (mcg)	0	0
Vitamin A (RAE) (mcg)	71.5	108
Vitamin E (mg)	2.4	0.5
Calcium (mg)	58.5	66
Iron (mg)	2.7	3.1
Magnesium (mg)	69	80
Potassium (mg)	790	988.4
Zinc (mg)	3	2.5
Sodium (mg)	40	111.5

Portion 1 Cup

Number of Exchanges

Traditional Recipe
2/3 non-starchy vegetable exchange
1 1/3 meat exchange
(1 high fat, 1/3 very lean)
2 1/2 fat exchange (PUFA)
1/3 starch exchange

Healthy Recipe
1 non-starchy vegetable exchange
2/3 meat exchange
(1/3 medium fat, 1/3 very lean)
1/3 starch exchange

Calories from Macronutrients

Protein Carbohydrates Fat

Traditional Recipe

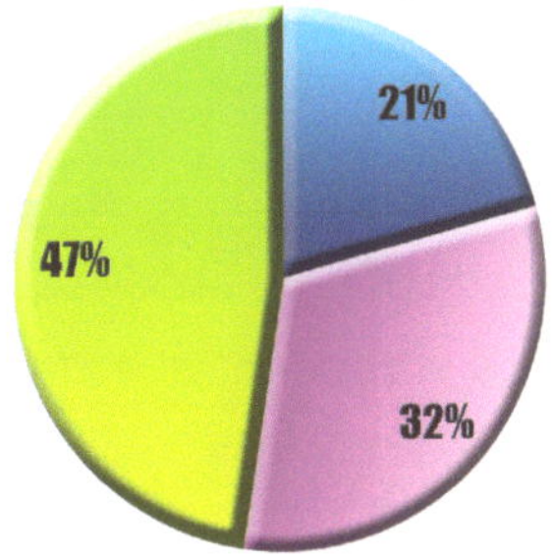

Healthy Recipe

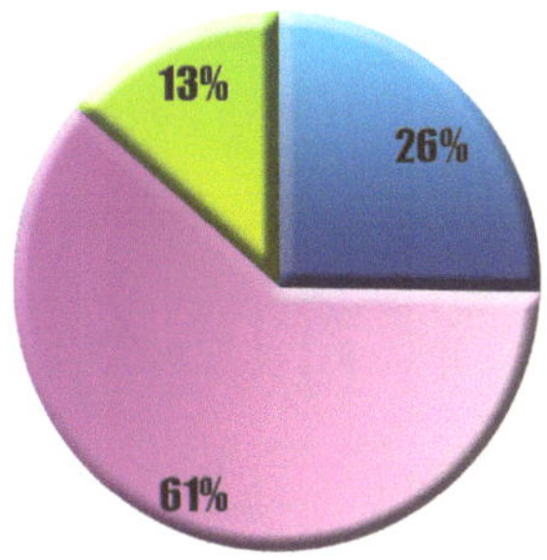

% Fiber Intake Compared to Average Daily Needs

Remaining Required Daily Consumed

Traditional Recipe

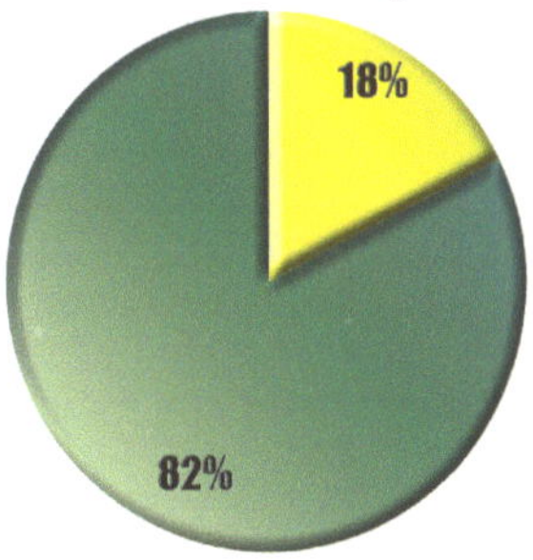

Healthy Recipe

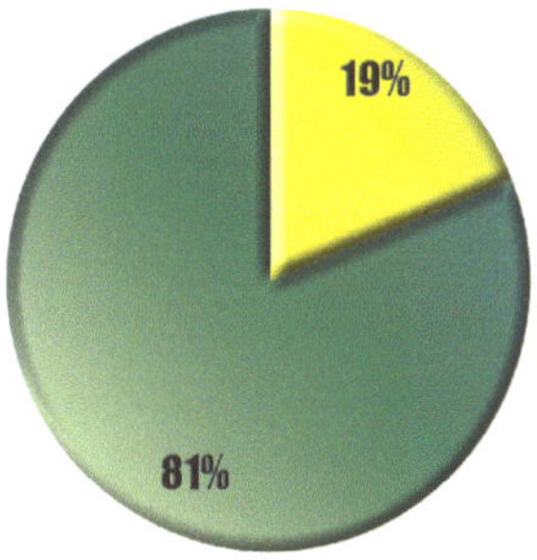

Recommended Portion Sizes & Meal Combinations

Traditional Recipe
(Calorie Controlled)

Men
2 1/4 cups of mosakaa kousa & Hummus
2 slices of small white pita bread

Women
1 1/2 cups of mosakaa kousa & Hummus
1 slice of small white pita bread

Healthy Recipe
(Calorie Controlled & Content Balanced)

Men
3 1/2 cups of mosakaa kousa & Hummus
2 slices of small whole wheat pita bread
1 cup of lowfat ayran

Women
2 cups of mosakaa kousa & Hummus
1 slice of small whole wheat pita bread
1 cup of lowfat ayran

Number of Exchanges in a Balanced Meal

Men
3 1/2 non-starchy vegetable exchange
2 meat exchange
(1 medium fat, 1 very lean)
1 starch exchange
2 grain exchange
1 milk exchange

Women
2 non-starchy vegetable exchange
1 1/3 meat exchange (2/3 medium fat, 2/3 very lean)
2/3 starch exchange
1 grain exchange
1 milk exchange

Everyday Side Dishes

Healthy Egg-Noodle Rice, 4 cups:

Ingredients:

2/3 cup Egg Noodles~48.6g

1 3/4 cups Short Rice~340g

2 Tbsp Corn Oil~31g

1 3/4 cups Water

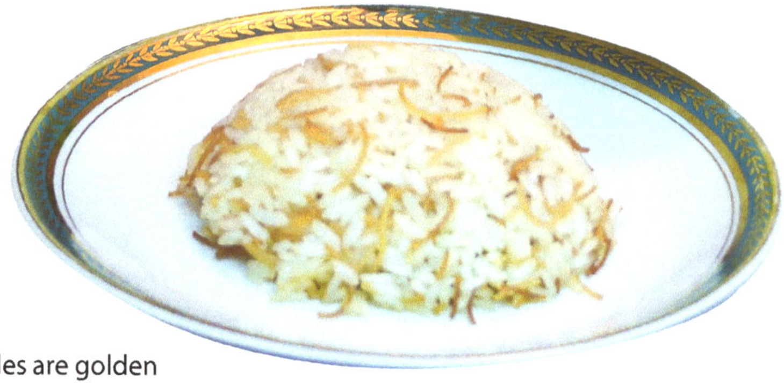

Method of Preparation:

- Wash rice under a running water until water is clear
- Soak rice in warm water for 20 minutes
- Heat cooking pan on a medium heat for 5 minutes
- Place egg-noodles and stir continuously until egg-noodles are golden
- Add rice and 1 cup of water; stir twice and cover for 10 minutes
- Add oil, reduce heat to low and continue to cook for 3 minutes
- Ready to serve

Calorie content per cup: 138.5

Number of Exchanges Per Serving: 1/3 Cup

1/2 polyunsaturated fat exchange

1 1/4 grain exchange

Healthy Dekous Eggplant, 4 cups:

Ingredients:

13 1/2 cups Eggplant~1286.4g

1/2 cup Fresh Chopped Cilantro~115.2 g

3 1/4 Tbsp Ground Garlic~39g

6 1/2 Tbsp Ground Cumin~19.2 g

2 3/4 Tbsp Olive Oil~38.4g

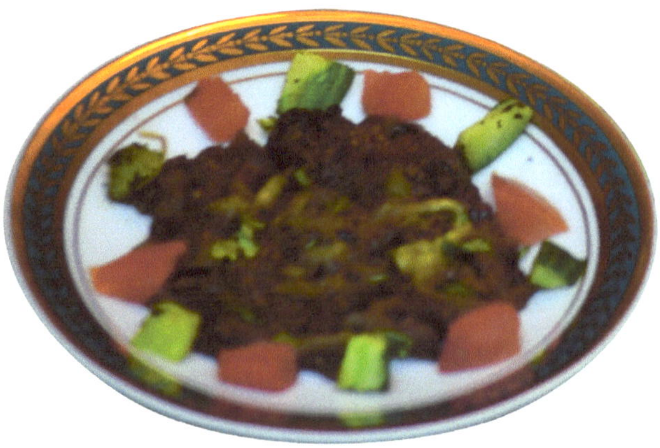

Method of Preparation:

- Preheat oven at medium heat
- Place eggplant in oven at medium heat for 10 minutes
- Peel grilled eggplants
- Mix eggplant, garlic, cumin, and cilantro together
- Garnish with olive oil
- Ready to serve

Note: The oil content is controlled in the healthy recipe when it is much higher in the traditional recipe.

Calorie Content per cup: 184

Number of Exchanges Per Serving: 1 Cup

3 1/3 non-starchy vegetable exchange

2 monounsaturated fat exchange

Healthy Yogurt Cucumber Salad, 4 cups:

Ingredients:

2 1/3 cups Lowfat Yogurt~580g

3 cups Chopped Cucumber~364g

1 1/3 tsp Ground Garlic~7.2g

5 tsp Peppermint Powder~2.4g

Method of Preparation:

- Mix ingredients together

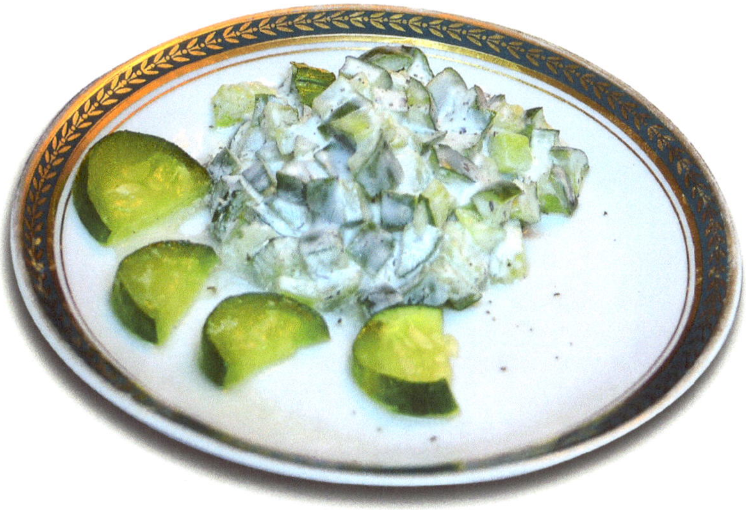

Calorie Content per cup: 117

Number of Exchanges Per Serving: 1 Cup

2/3 milk exchange

3/4 non-starchy vegetable exchange

Healthy Green Salad, 4 cups:

Select your favorite green vegetables and drizzle each cup with 1 teaspoon of olive oil

Healthy Lowfat Ayran, 1 cup:

Ingredients:

2 2/3 cup lowfat Yogurt~652g

1 cup Water

Method of Preparation:

- Mix together

Optional: Add 2 teaspoons of ground garlic

Calorie Content per cup: 102

Number of Exchanges Per Serving: 1 Cup

1 milk exchange

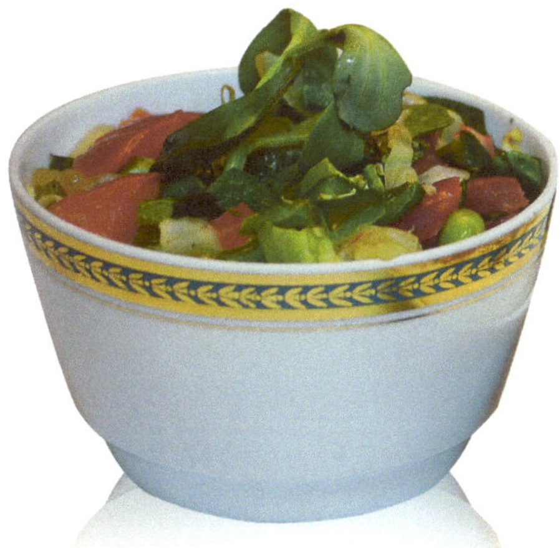

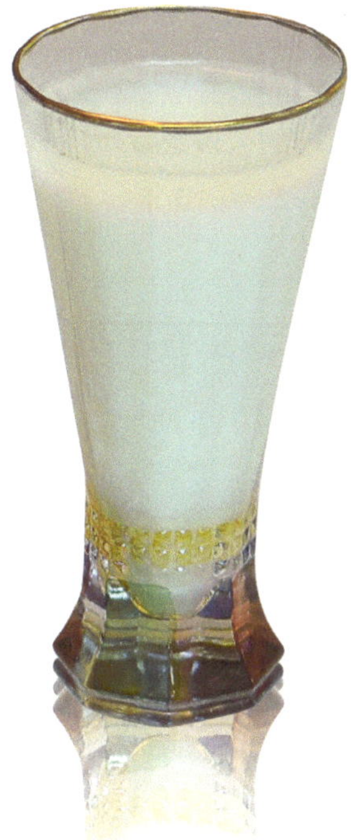

Serving: 1 Cup
(Examples)

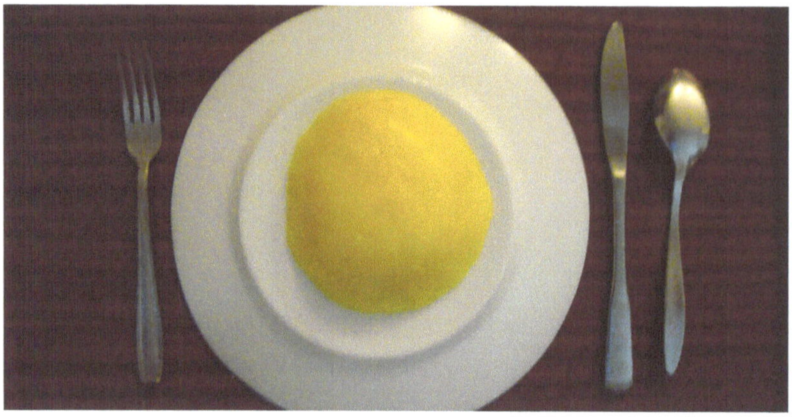

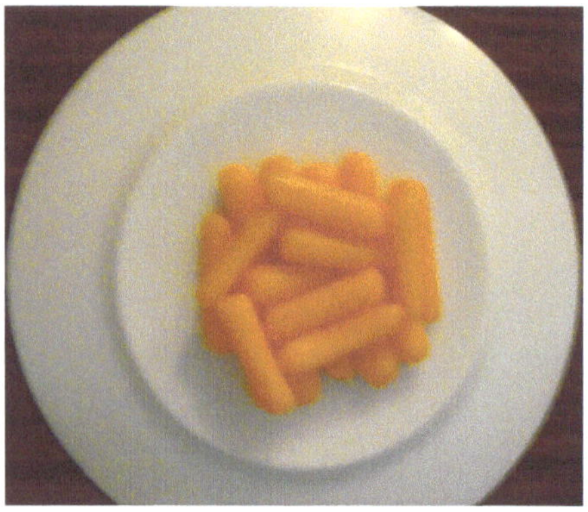

1 cup of fresh carrots

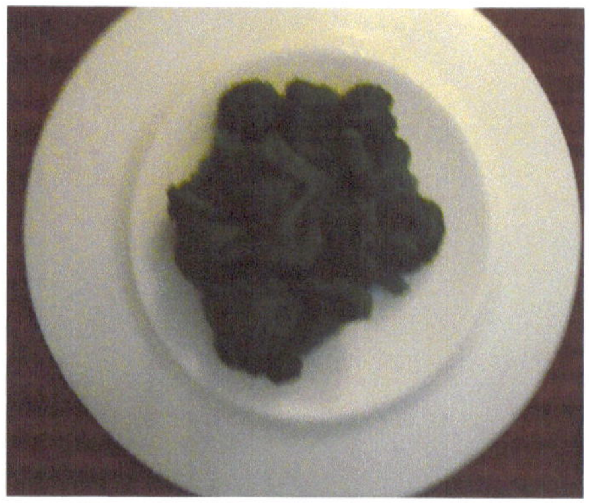

1 cup of cooked broccoli

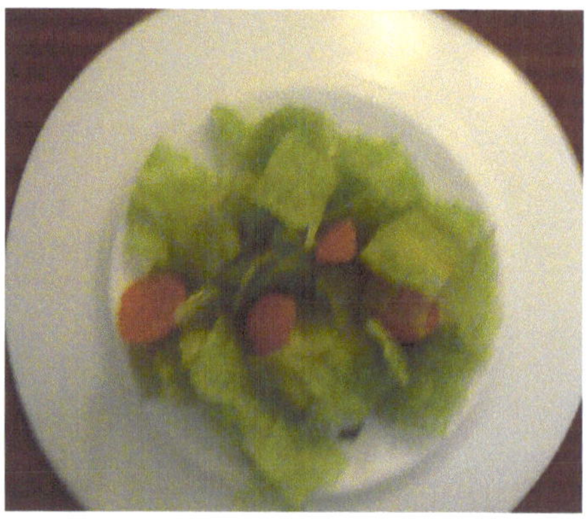

1 cup of fresh salad

Bread Servings & By-Products

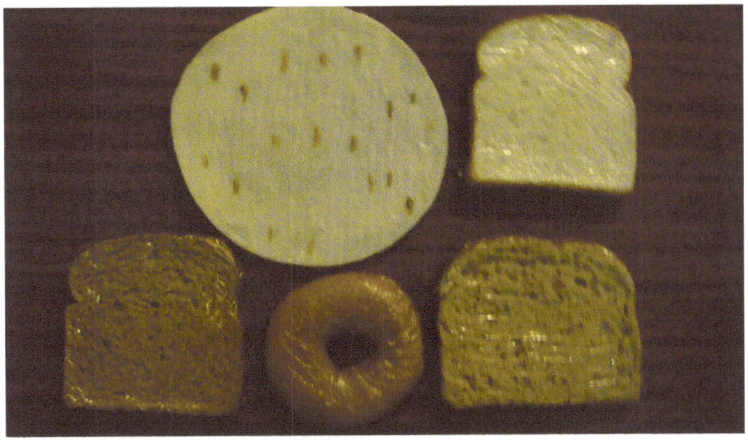

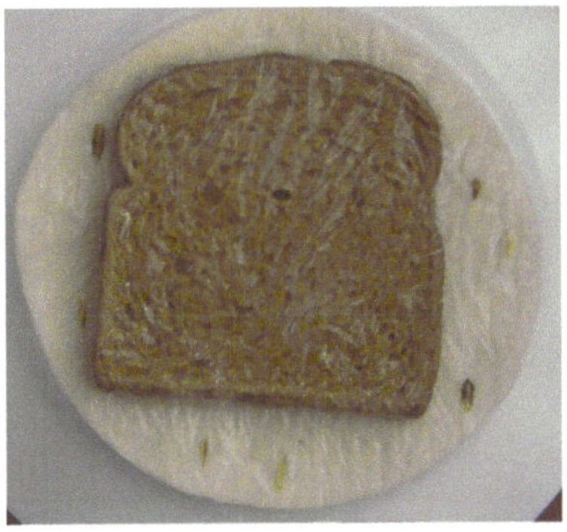

Slice of Bread

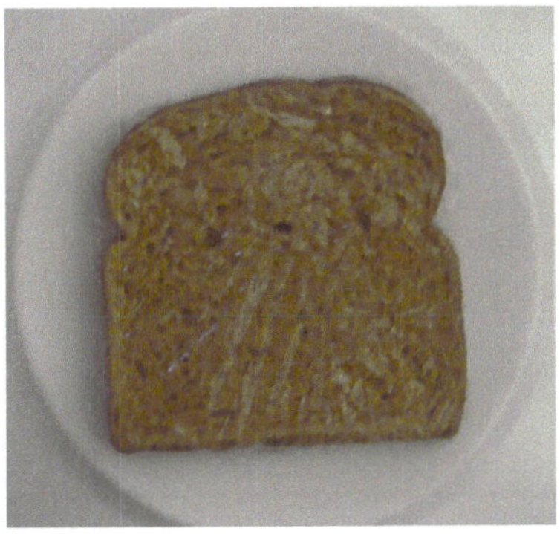

Slice of Toast: 28 grams

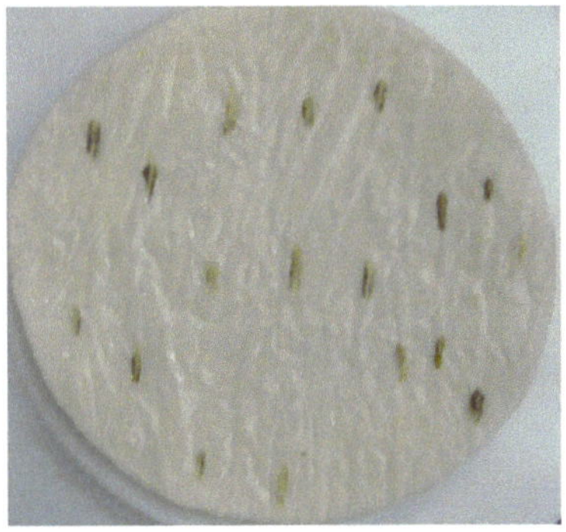

Slice of Medium Pita Bread
Diameter: 30 cm/28 grams

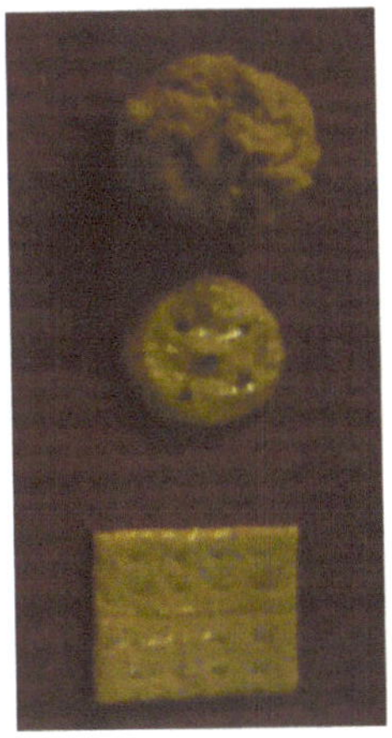

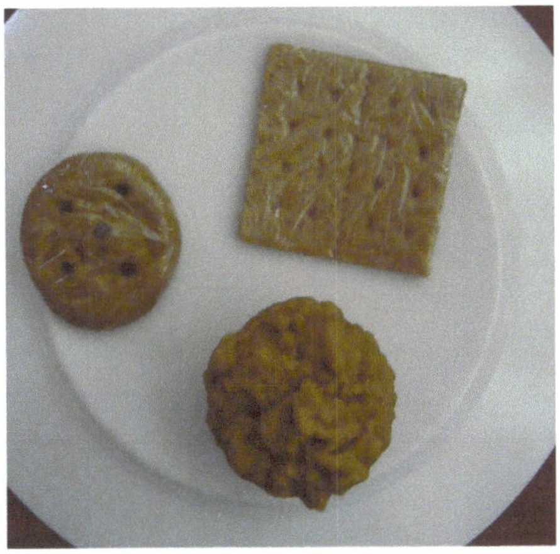

One Cracker

One Cookie

One Cup Cake

A piece of Cake
2 square/5 cm

Width: 5 cm
Height: 5 cm

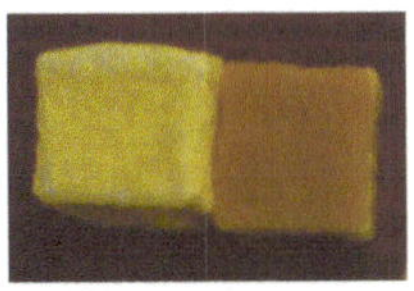

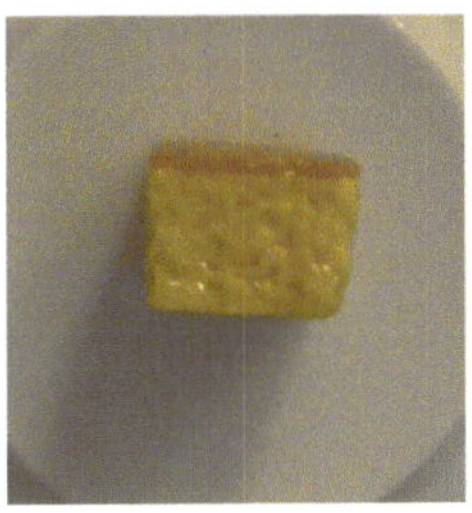

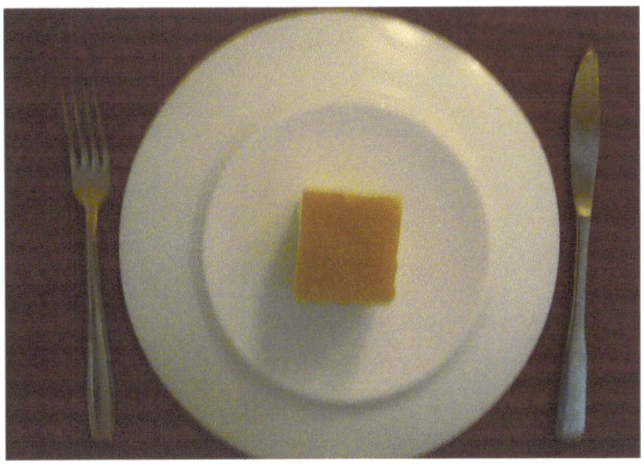

Estimated Calorie Needs per Day by Age, Gender, and Physical Activity:

(United States of Agriculture: Center for Nutrition Policy and Promotion, Released on 1/31/2011) Physical Activity

Physical Activity

Gender	Age (Years)	Sedentary	Moderately Active	Active
Child (female& male)	2-3	1000-1200	1000-1400	1000-1400
Female	4-8	1200-1400	1400-1600	1400-1800
	9-13	1400-1600	1600-2000	1800-2200
	14-18	1800	2000	2400
	19-30	1800-2000	2000-2200	2400
	31-50	1800	2000	2200
	51+	1600	1800	2000-2200
Male	4-8	1200-1400	1400-1600	1600-1800
	9-13	1600-2000	1800-2200	2000-2600
	14-18	2000-2400	2400-2800	2800-3200
	19-30	2400-2600	2600-2800	3000
	31-50	2200-2400	2400-2600	2800-3000
	51+	2000-2200	2200-2400	2400-2800

Dietary Reference Intakes (DRIs): Recommended Intakes for Individuals: Carbohydrates, Fiber, Fat, Fatty Acids, and Protein.

Source: Institute of Medicine, Food and Nutrition Board, "Dietary Reference Intakes for Energy, Carbohydrates, Fiber, Fat, Protein, and Amino Acids." Washigton, D.C.: National Academy Press, 2002.

Life Stage Group	Carbohydrate (g/day)	Fiber (g/day)	Fat (g/day)	Omega 6 Fatty Acid (g/day)	Omega 3 Fatty Acid (g/day)	Protein (g/kg/day)	(g/day)
Infant							
0-6 months	60 *	ND	31*	4.4*	0.5*	1.52*	9.1*
6-12 months	95*	ND	30*	4.6*	0.5*	1.5	13.5
Children							
1-3 years	130	19*	ND	7*	0.7*	1.1	13
4-8 years	130	25*	ND	10*	0.9*	0.95	19
Males							
9-13 years	130	31*	ND	12*	1.2*	0.95	34
14-18 years	130	38*	ND	16*	1.6*	0.85	52
19-30 years	130	38*	ND	17*	1.6*	0.8	56
31-50 years	130	38*	ND	17*	1.6*	0.8	56
51-70 years	130	30*	ND	14*	1.6*	0.8	56
>70 years	130	30*	ND	14*	1.6*	0.8	56
Female							
9-13 years	130	26*	ND	10*	1*	0.95	34
14-18 years	130	26*	ND	11*	1.1*	0.85	46
19-30 years	130	25*	ND	12*	1.1*	0.8	46
31-50 years	130	25*	ND	12*	1.1*	0.8	46
51-70 years	130	21*	ND	11*	1.1*	0.8	46
>70 years	130	21*	ND	11*	1.1	0.8	46
Pregnancy							
14-18 years	175	28*	ND	13*	1.4*	1.1	71
19-30 years	175	28*	ND	13*	1.4*	1.1	71
31-50 years	175	28*	ND	13*	1.4*	1.1	71
Lactation							
14-18 years	210	29*	ND	13*	1.3*	1.1	71
19-30 years	210	29*	ND	13*	1.3*	1.1	71
31-50 years	210	29*	ND	13*	1.3*	1.1	71

ND: Not Determined

*Values are Adequate Intake

Dietary Reference Intakes (DRIs): Recommended Intakes for Individuals: Carbohydrates, Fiber, Fat, Fatty Acids, and Protein.

Source: Institute of Medicine, Food and Nutrition Board, "Dietary Reference Intakes for Energy, Carbohydrates, Fiber, Fat, Protein, and Amino Acids." Washigton, D.C.: National Academy Press, 2002.

Life Stage Group	Carbohydrate (g/day)	Fiber (g/day)	Fat (g/day)	Omega 6 Fatty Acid (g/day)	Omega 3 Fatty Acid (g/day)	Protein (g/kg/day)	Protein (g/day)
Infant							
0-6 months	60 *	ND	31*	4.4*	0.5*	1.52*	9.1*
6-12 months	95*	ND	30*	4.6*	0.5*	1.5	13.5
Children							
1-3 years	130	19*	ND	7*	0.7*	1.1	13
4-8 years	130	25*	ND	10*	0.9*	0.95	19
Males							
9-13 years	130	31*	ND	12*	1.2*	0.95	34
14-18 years	130	38*	ND	16*	1.6*	0.85	52
19-30 years	130	38*	ND	17*	1.6*	0.8	56
31-50 years	130	38*	ND	17*	1.6*	0.8	56
51-70 years	130	30*	ND	14*	1.6*	0.8	56
>70 years	130	30*	ND	14*	1.6*	0.8	56
Female							
9-13 years	130	26*	ND	10*	1*	0.95	34
14-18 years	130	26*	ND	11*	1.1*	0.85	46
19-30 years	130	25*	ND	12*	1.1*	0.8	46
31-50 years	130	25*	ND	12*	1.1*	0.8	46
51-70 years	130	21*	ND	11*	1.1*	0.8	46
>70 years	130	21*	ND	11*	1.1	0.8	46
Pregnancy							
14-18 years	175	28*	ND	13*	1.4*	1.1	71
19-30 years	175	28*	ND	13*	1.4*	1.1	71
31-50 years	175	28*	ND	13*	1.4*	1.1	71
Lactation							
14-18 years	210	29*	ND	13*	1.3*	1.1	71
19-30 years	210	29*	ND	13*	1.3*	1.1	71
31-50 years	210	29*	ND	13*	1.3*	1.1	71

ND: Not Determined
*Values are Adequate Intake

Dietary Reference Intakes: Recommended Intakes and Adequate Intakes for Individuals: Vitamins and Minerals:

Sources: Trumbo, P.,A., Yates, S. Schilcker, M. Poos. "Dietary Reference Intakes: Vitamin A, Vitamin K, Arsenic, Boron, Chromium, Copper, Iodine, Iron, Manganese, Molybdenum, Nickel, Silicon, Vanadium, and Zinc." Journal of the American Dietetic Association 101, no.3 (2001) 294-301.

	Life Stage Group	Thiamin (mg/day)	Riboflavin (mg/day)	Niacin (mg/day)	Vitamin B6 (mg/day)	Vitamin B12 (mcg/day)	Folate (DFE) (mcg/day)	Vitamin C (mg/day)	Vitamin D (mcg/day)	Vitamin A (RAE) (mcg/day)	Vitamin E Calcium (mg/day) (mg/day)	Iron (mg/day)	Magnesium (mg/day)	Potassium (mg/day)	Zinc (mg/day)	Sodium (mg/day)
Infant																
0-6 months	0.2*	0.3*	2*	0.1*	0.4*	65*	40*	5*	400*	4*	210*	0.27*	30*	0.4	2*	0.12
6-12 months	0.3*	0.4*	4*	0.3*	0.5*	80*	50*	5*	500*	5*	270*	11	75*	0.7	3	0.37
Children																
1-3 years	0.5	0.5	6	0.5	0.9	150	15	5*	300	6	500*	7	80	3	3	1
4-8 years	0.6	0.8	8	0.5	1.2	200	25	5*	400	7	800*	10	130	3.8	5	1.2
Males																
9-13 years	1	0.9	12	1	1.8	300	45	5*	600	11	1300*	8	240	4.5	8	1.5
14-18 years	1.3	1.3	16	1.3	2.4	400	75	5*	900	15	1300*	11	410	4.7	11	1.5
19-30 years	1.3	1.3	16	1.3	2.4	400	90	5*	900	15	1000*	8	400	4.7	11	1.5
31-50 years	1.3	1.3	16	1.3	2.4	400	90	5*	900	15	1000*	8	420	4.7	11	1.5
51-70 years	1.7	1.3	16	1.7	2.4	400	90	10*	900	15	1200*	8	420	4.7	11	1.3
>70 years	1.7	1.3	16	1.7	2.4	400	90	15*	900	15	1200*	8	420	4.7	11	1.2
Female																
9-13 years	1	0.9	12	1	1.8	300	45	5*	600	11	1300*	8	240	4.5	8	1.5
14-18 years	1.2	1	14	1.2	2.4	400	65	5*	700	15	1300*	15	360	4.7	9	1.5
19-30 years	1.3	1.1	14	1.3	2.4	400	75	5*	700	15	1000	18	310	4.7	8	1.5
31-50 years	1.3	1.1	14	1.3	2.4	400	75	5*	700	15	1000	18	320	4.7	8	1.5
51-70 years	1.5	1.1	14	1.5	2.4	400	75	10*	700	15	1200*	8	320	4.7	8	1.3
>70 years	1.5	1.1	14	1.5	2.4	400	75	15*	700	15	1200*	8	320	4.7	8	1.2
Pregnancy																
14-18 years	1.9	1.4	18	1.9	2.6	600	80	5*	750	15	1300*	27	400	4.7	13	
19-30 years	1.9	1.4	18	1.9	2.6	600	85	5*	770	15	1000*	27	350	4.7	11	
31-50 years	1.9	1.4	18	1.9	2.6	600	85	5*	770	15	1000*	27	360	4.7	11	
Lactation																
14-18 years	2	1.6	17	2	2.8	500	115	5*	1200	19	1300*	10	360	5.1	14	
19-30 years	2	1.6	17	2	2.8	500	120	5*	1300	19	1300*	9	310	5.1	12	
31-50 years	2	1.6	17	2	2.8	500	120	5*	1300	19	1300*	9	320	5.1	12	

ND: Not Determined

*Values are Adequate Intake

Metric Conversion Guide

Volume	US UNITS	CANADIAN METRIC	AUSTRALIAN METRIC
	1/4 teaspoon	1 ml	1 ml
	1/2 teaspoon	2 ml	2 ml
	1 teaspoon	5 ml	5 ml
	1 tablespoon	15 ml	20 ml
	1/4 cup	50 ml	60 ml
	1/3 cup	75 ml	80 ml
	1/2 cup	125 ml	125 ml
	2/3 cup	150 ml	170 ml
	3/4 cup	175 ml	190 ml
	1 cup	250 ml	250 ml
	1 quart	1 liter	1 liter

Weight	US UNITS	CANADIAN METRIC	AUSTRALIAN METRIC
	2 ounces	55 grams	60 grams
	3 ounces	85 grams	90 grams
	4 ounces (1/4 pound)	115 grams	125 grams
	8 ounces (1/2 pounds)	225 grams	225 grams
	16 ounces (1 pound)	455 grams	500 grams
	1 pound	455 grams	1/2 kilogram

Temperature

Fahrenheit	Celsius
32	0
212	100
250	120
275	140
300	150
325	160
350	180
375	190
400	200
425	220
450	230
475	240
500	260

NOTE: The recipes in this book were developed and tested using US units for Volume and Canadian Metric for Weight. When covering recipes some variations in quality may be noted.

Acknowledgments

To the strong man, who taught me patience and dedication
To the skillful man, who educated me on hard-work and determination
To the caring man, who coached me with plenty of devotion
To the loveable man, whom I run out of words to express my appreciation
To you, my **Father**, *I stand here grateful with infinite love and obligation*
Because of you, I am proud; your sacrifice made me reach this destination
Baba Amir, *I will always need you and my thanks have no limitations*

Lifetime of giving
Days and nights without sleeping
Raising, teaching, and always loving
Here I stand, hopefully as you were wishing
If I used all the world's languages to thank you, some would be missing
Today, I thank you ***Mama*** *for every minute you spent helping accomplish my work*
For the efforts you put into saving my time & for wiping my tears when I was stressed
For strengthening me, when I felt it was too hard
Thanks for having me in your heart; just to please me with your tears or with your smiles
Mama Rafat, *my apology, If I fail to give you back, I only hope that you are proud*

I would like to take time and thank the person who suggested this research
This person has helped make every obstacle a new successful step forward
I owe him so much for motivating and inspiring me
At the beginning of my career, he believed in me
and encouraged me to keep going, and to always stand
Dr. Hussam Trabusli, *a successful Bariatric Surgeon*
whom God has blessed me to work and partner with
I am grateful for you allowing me to introduce myself to society
as a Professional Pharmacist and Dietitian; a million thanks!

As we grew up, we learned that
"there is always a candle burning to lighten our pathway to success"
I realized the truth behind this saying once I met this person
My professor, my advisor, and my mentor
Dr. Fatma Huffman
Thank you ***Dr. Huffman*** *for always being there with open hands to help. You never hesitated to extend your love, care, support, and knowledge during my Undergraduate and the stressful Post-graduate studies in Nutrition.*
Today, I thank you ***Dr. Huffman*** *for every minute you spent guiding, advising, and reviewing my work*
My respect, appreciation, and gratitude!.

Three stars brightens my days of darkness
Three stars lightened the road of my sadness
My three brothers, ***Feras***, ***Tarek***, *and* ***Wael***
I thank you ***Feras*** *for every tiring night you spent with me while I was doing this work*

I thank you for your motivational jokes that always made me laugh,
even when I was about to give up and cry
I thank you **Tarek** for the effort you repeated every day to help me
continue the work. I thank you wonderful man for being a joyful part of my life
Wael, the little star that gives most of the light, I thank you for always being there
to motivate and take care of me. I thank you for every effort you put into
easing the barriers, which caused obstacles to become blocks of success, I thank you!

A blessing by God
A beautiful moon in my life…my sister, **Haya**
You spice up my life with your fury or with your smile
You are always there, even when I don't ask
I thank you **Haya** for helping me to continue the work during my days of sickness
Your attempts touched my heart. Your motivation and your inspiration were such a great part of my persistence to finish this work, I love you!

The beautiful flower in my life, my grandpa, **Jedo Raif**
A wise man who is always there to inspire and advise
Thank you for the love and care that you always share
Thank you for providing me with a collection of cooking books to help me
My knowledgeable **Jedo**, may God bless you and protect you always
Thank you for being a great Grandfather!

Thank you my great people for sharing with me your cooking methods
and for providing me with original cookbooks from different Middle Eastern countries
Thank you **Mrs. Nahla Alessa** from Kuwait, **Mrs. Nahed Sagherji** from Syria, **Mrs. Susan Hamdoun** from KSA, **Mrs. Hend Majed** from Iraq
And a special thanks to the hands of that lady who worked behind the scene
and was willing to help and support in my cooking endeavors,
Mrs. Amena Al-Herafi, one of the most famous and historical cooks in Damascus-Syria.
You never hesitated to share your cooking secrets that help save time and guaranteed
pleasurable results, thank you!

I thank my **patients** and **clients** for supporting my absence during the days of my stay in the United States of America to help complete this project. I am very grateful for the difference you all made in my life. The satisfactory results you experience are success-markers to my career. The great friendships we have built together add new meaning to my life. Thanks to each and every one of you, **the family of my clinic, Fat2Slim**.

Last but not least, I thank you my **special friends** and the **VJ Publishing House, LLC team**.
Your emotional support and motivation were invisible reasons to accomplish this work during the last steps and during the most stressful time! My special thanks with pure love!

~Racha Sankar~

REFERENCES

References

1: Abdulbari, Bener, and Kamal Abdulaziz A. Growth patterns of Qatari school children and adolescents aged 6-18 years. Index Medicus for South-East Asia Region (IMSEAR), 2005, 23(3): 250-8.

2: Al-Hazzaa , Hazzaz M., and Amani A. Al-Rasheedi. Adiposity and physical activity levels among preschool children in Jeddah, Saudi Arabia. Saudi Medical Journal,2007, 28(5): 766-773.

3: Al Orifan, Faisal H., Hanan E. Badr, et al.Obesity and Cardiovascular Risk Factors in Kuwaiti Adults. KUWAIT MEDICAL JOURNAL,2007, 39(2): 162-166.

4: Al-Othaimeen, A I, M Al-Nozha, et al. Obesity: an emerging problem in Saudi Arabia. Analysis of data from the National Nutrition Survey. Eastern Mediterranean health journal, 2007, 13(2):441-448.

5: Al-Nozha , Mansour M., Yacoub Y. Al-Mazrou, et al. Obesity in Saudi Arabia. Saudi Medical Journal, 2005, 5(26): 824-829.

6: Al-Raees, Ghada Y. , et al. "Prevalence of overweight and obesity among children aged 2–5 years in Bahrain: A comparison between two reference standards. International Journal of Pediatric Obesity, 2009, 4(4):414-416.

7: Al Sabbah, H., C. Vereecken, et al, et al. Associations of overweight and of weight dissatisfaction among Palestinian adolescents: findings from the national study of Palestinian schoolchildren (HBSC-WBG2004). Journal of Human Nutrition and Dietetics, 2009, 22(1):40–49.

8: Asfar, Taghrid, Balsam Ahmad, et al. Self-rated health and its determinants among adults in Syria: a model from the Middle East.BMC Public Health, 2007, 7(177): 1471-2458.

9: El Mouzan, Mohammad I., Peter J. Foster , et al. Prevalence of overweight and obesity in Saudi children and adolescents. Ann Saudi Med, 2010, 30(3):203–208.

10: El-Hazmi, Mohsen A.F., and Arjumand S. Warsy. THE PREVALENCE OF OBESITY AND OVERWEIGHT IN 1-18-YEAR-OLD SAUDI CHILDREN. Annals of Saudi Medicine, 2002, 22(5-6):303-307.

11: El-Bayoumy, Ibrahim. Et al. Prevalence of Obesity Among Adolescents (10 to 14 Years) in Kuwait. Asia Pac J Public Health,2009, 21(2):153-159

12: Fazah, Abdallah, Christophe Jacob, et al. Activity, inactivity and quality of life among Lebanese adolescents." Pediatrics International, 2010, 52(4): 573–578.

13: Husseini, Abdullatif, Niveen ME Abu-Rmeileh, et al. Cardiovascular diseases, diabetes mellitus, and cancer in the occupied Palestinian territory. THE LANCET, 2009, 373(9668):1041–1049.

14: Khader, Yousef, and Anwar Batieha, et all. Obesity in Jordan: Prevalence, Associated Factors, Comorbidities, and Change in Prevalence over Ten Years. Metabolic Syndrome and Related Disorders,2008, 6(2): 113-120.

15: Khader, Yousef , et al. Overweight and Obesity Among School Children in Jordan: Prevalence and Associated Factors. MATERNAL AND CHILD HEALTH JOURNAL,2009, 13(3):424-431.

16: Lafta, Riyadh K, et al. Childhood obesity in Iraq: prevalence and possible risk factors.Ann Saudi Med, 2005, 25(5):389-393.

17: Malik, M., and A. Bakir. Prevalence of overweight and obesity among children in the United Arab Emirates. Obesity Reviews, 2007, 8(1):15–20.

18: Martorell R et al. Obesity in women from developing countries. European journal of clinical nutrition, 2000, 54(3):247-52.

19: M.F., Fouad, and Rastam S, et al. Prevalence of obesity and its associated factors in Aleppo, Syria. Prevention and Control, 2006, 2(2):85–94.

20: Motlagh, Bahareh, Martin O'Donnell, et al. Prevalence of cardiovascular risk factors in the Middle East: a systematic review. European Journal of Preventive Cardiology, 2009, 16(3):268-280.

21: Nasreddine, L. Adolescent obesity in Syria: prevalence and associated factors. Child: Care, Health and Development, 2010, 36(3):404-413.

22: Ng, S. W., S. Zaghloul, et al, et al. The prevalence and trends of overweight, obesity and nutrition-related non-communicable diseases in the Arabian Gulf States. Obesity Review,2011, 12(1):1-13.

23: Osman YF et al. Progression of obesity among Seeb school children in Oman. A preliminary study. Saudi Medical Journal, 2004, 25(12):2038–2040.

24: Salazar-Martinez, Eduardo, et al. Overweight and Obesity Status among Adolescents from Mexico and Egypt. Archived of Medical Research, 2006, 37(4): 535–542.

25: Saadi, Hussein, S. George Carruthers, et al.Prevalence of diabetes mellitus and its complications in a population-based sample in Al Ain, United Arab Emirates. Diabetes Research and Clinical Practice, 2007, 78(3):369–377.

26: Sibai, Abla Mehio, Nahla Hwalla, et al. Prevalence and Covariates of Obesity inLebanon: Findings from the First Epidemiological Study. Obesity Research,2003, 11: 1353–1361.

27: YA, Raja'a, et al. Overweight and Obesity among Schoolchildren in Sana'a City, Yemen. Ann Nutr Metab, 2005, 49(5):342–345.

28 : Zubaid, M., C.G. Suresh, et al. "Differential Distribution of Risk Factors and Outcome of Acute Coronary Syndrome in Kuwait: Three Years' Experience.Med Princ Pract, 2004, 13:63–68.

We hoped you enjoyed this VJ Publishing House, LLC. Publication.
If you would like additional information, please contact:

VJ
PUBLISHING HOUSE, LLC.

VJ Publishing House, LLC.
320 S. Flamingo Road, Suite #305
Pembroke Pines, Florida 33027
(Toll free) 888-567-6582
Fax: 954-404-8363

Visit our website at
www.vjpublishinghouse.com

If you would like to share how this recipe book helped or encourage you, or to book RPh, D. Racha Sankar for a group or organization engagement/workshop/book signing etc., you can contact her at: racha@vjpublishinghouse.com

www.ingramcontent.com/pod-product-compliance
Lightning Source LLC
LaVergne TN
LVHW071241210926
848486LV00007B/320
9781939236012